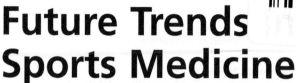

Future Trends Sports Medicine

Guest Editor

SCOTT A. RODEO, MD

CLINICS IN
SPORTS MEDICINE

www.sportsmed.theclinics.com

Consulting Editor
MARK D. MILLER, MD

January 2009 • Volume 28 • Number 1

SAUNDERS an imprint of ELSEVIER, Inc.

W.B. SAUNDERS COMPANY

A Division of Elsevier Inc.

1600 John F. Kennedy Blvd. • Suite 1800 • Philadelphia, Pennsylvania 19103

http://www.theclinics.com

CLINICS IN SPORTS MEDICINE Volume 28, Number 1
January 2009 ISSN 0278-5919, ISBN-13: 978-1-4377-0542-3, ISBN-10: 1-4377-0542-1

Editor: Ruth Malwitz

Clinics in Sports Medicine (ISSN 0278-5919) is published quarterly by Elsevier Inc., 360 Park Avenue South, New York, NY 10010-1710. Months of publication are January, April, July, and October. Business and Editorial Offices: 1600 John F. Kennedy Blvd., Suite 1800, Philadelphia, PA 19103-2899. Customer Service Offices: 6277 Sea Harbor Drive, Orlando, FL 32887-4800. Periodicals postage paid at New York, NY, and additional mailing offices. Subscription prices are $253.00 per year (US individuals), $393.00 per year (US institutions), $127.00 per year (US students), $286.00 per year (Canadian individuals), $475.00 per year (Canadian institutions), $177.00 (Canadian students), $347.00 per year (foreign individuals), $475.00 per year (foreign institutions), and $177.00 per year (foreign students). Foreign air speed delivery is included in all *Clinics* subscription prices. All prices are subject to change without notice. **POSTMASTER:** Send address changes to *Clinics in Sports Medicine*, Elsevier Periodicals Customer Service, 11830 Westline Industrial Drive, St. Louis, MO 63146. Customer Service (orders, claims, online, change of address): Elsevier Periodicals Customer Service, 11830 Westline Industrial Drive, St. Louis, MO 63146. Tel: 1-800-654-2452 (U.S. and Canada); 314-453-7041 (outside U.S. and Canada). Fax: 314-453-5170. E-mail: journalscustomerservice-usa@elsevier.com (for print support); journalsonlinesupport-usa@elsevier.com (for online support).

Reprints. For copies of 100 or more of articles in this publication, please contact the Commercial Reprints Department, Elsevier Inc., 360 Park Avenue South, New York, NY 10010-1710. Tel.: 212-633-3812; Fax: 212-462-1935; E-mail: reprints@elsevier.com.

Clinics in Sports Medicine is covered in *MEDLINE/PubMed (Index Medicus) Current Contents/Clinical Medicine, Excerpta Medica,* and *ISI/Biomed.*

Printed and bound by CPI Group (UK) Ltd, Croydon, CR0 4YY

Transferred to Digital Print 2011

Contributors

CONSULTING EDITOR

MARK D. MILLER, MD
S. Ward Casscells Professor of Orthopaedic Surgery, Department of Orthopaedic Surgery; Director, Division of Sports Medicine, University of Virginia Health System, Charlottesville, Virginia

GUEST EDITOR

SCOTT A. RODEO, MD
Chief, Sports Medicine and Shoulder Service, The Hospital for Special Surgery; Professor of Orthopaedic Surgery (Academic Track), Weill Medical College of Cornell University; Attending Orthopaedic Surgeon, The Hospital for Special Surgery; Attending Surgeon (Orthopaedic Surgery), The New York-Presbyterian Hospital; Assistant Scientist, Department of Research, The Hospital for Special Surgery; Associate Team Physician, New York Giants Football, New York, New York

AUTHORS

BRANDON R. BLACK, MD
Musculoskeletal MRI Fellow, The Hospital for Special Surgery, Weill Medical College of Cornell University, New York, New York

PIETER BUMA, PhD
Orthopedic Research Laboratory, Radboud University Nijmegen Medical Centre, Nijmegen, The Netherlands

WILLIAM CATES, PT, DPT, ES
The Hospital for Special Surgery, Sports Rehabilitation and Performance Center, New York, New York

JOHN CAVANAUGH, PT, Med, ATC
Clinical Supervisor, The Hospital for Special Surgery, Sports Rehabilitation and Performance Center, New York, New York

LE ROY CHONG, MD
MRI Research Fellow, The Hospital for Special Surgery, Weill Medical College of Cornell University, New York, New York

M. CITAK, MD
Sports Medicine and Shoulder Service, The Hospital for Special Surgery, New York, New York

RYAN DELLAMAGGIORA, MD
Department of Orthopaedic Surgery, University of Southern California, Keck School of Medicine, Healthcare Consultation Center, Los Angeles, California

FREDDIE H. FU, MD
Chairman, Department of Orthopaedic Surgery, University of Pittsburgh Medical Center, Pittsburgh, Pennsylvania

LAWRENCE V. GULOTTA, MD
Chief Resident in Orthopaedic Surgery, The Hospital for Special Surgery, Weill Medical College of Cornell University, New York, New York

GERJON HANNINK, PhD
Orthopedic Research Laboratory, Radboud University Nijmegen Medical Centre, Nijmegen, The Netherlands

JOHNNY HUARD, PhD
Henry J. Mankin Professor and Vice Chair for Research, Department of Orthopaedic Surgery, University of Pittsburgh Medical Center; Stem Cell Research Center, Children's Hospital of Pittsburgh, Rangos Research Center; Professor, Department of Microbiology and Molecular Genetics; Department of Bioengineering, University of Pittsburgh, Pittsburgh, Pennsylvania

D. KENDOFF, MD, PhD
Sports Medicine and Shoulder Service, The Hospital for Special Surgery, New York, New York

MARK LOVELL, PhD
Professor of Orthopedic Surgery, UPMC Sports Medicine Concussion Program, University of Pittsburgh Medical Center, Department of Orthopaedic Surgery, Pittsburgh, Pennsylvania

HELEN H. LU, PhD
Department of Biomedical Engineering, Biomaterials and Interface Tissue Engineering Laboratory, Columbia University, New York, New York

BERT R. MANDELBAUM, MD
Santa Monica Orthopedic and Sports Medicine Foundation, Los Angeles, California

TIMOTHY R. McADAMS, MD
Stanford University, Department of Orthopaedic Surgery, Palo Alto, California

ALLAN MISHRA, MD
Clinical Assistant Professor, Department of Orthopedic Surgery, Menlo Medical Clinic, Stanford University Medical Center, Menlo Park, California

KAI MITHOEFER, MD
Harvard Vanguard Orthopedics and Sports Medicine, Harvard Medical School, Boston, Massachusetts

KRISTEN L. MOFFAT, MS
Department of Biomedical Engineering, Biomaterials and Interface Tissue Engineering Laboratory, Columbia University, New York, New York

MARTHA M. MURRAY, MD
Assistant Professor of Orthopaedic Surgery, Harvard Medical School; Orthopaedic Surgeon, Children's Hospital of Boston, Boston, Massachusetts

A.D. PEARLE, MD
Sports Medicine and Shoulder Service, The Hospital for Special Surgery, New York, New York

HOLLIS G. POTTER, MD
Chief, Magnetic Resonance Imaging; Director of Research, Department of Radiology and Imaging, The Hospital for Special Surgery; Professor of Radiology, Weill Medical College of Cornell University, New York, New York

ANDRES J. QUINTERO, MD
Stem Cell Research Center, Children's Hospital of Pittsburgh, Rangos Research Center; Department of Orthopaedic Surgery, University of Pittsburgh Medical Center, Pittsburgh, Pennsylvania

SCOTT A. RODEO, MD
Chief, Sports Medicine and Shoulder Service, The Hospital for Special Surgery; Professor of Orthopaedic Surgery (Academic Track), Weill Medical College of Cornell University; Attending Orthopaedic Surgeon, The Hospital for Special Surgery; Attending Surgeon (Orthopaedic Surgery), The New York-Presbyterian Hospital; Assistant Scientist, Department of Research, The Hospital for Special Surgery; Associate Team Physician, New York Giants Football, New York, New York

JASON M. SCOPP, MD
Peninsula Orthopedic Associates, Salisbury, Maryland

SUKETU VAISHNAV, MD
Resident Physician, Department of Orthopaedic Surgery, University of Southern California, Keck School of Medicine, LAC+USC Medical Center, Los Angeles, California

C. THOMAS VANGSNESS, Jr., MD
Professor of Orthopaedics, Department of Orthopaedic Surgery, University of Southern California, Keck School of Medicine, Healthcare Consultation Center, Los Angeles, California

TONY G. van TIENEN, MD, PhD
Orthopedic Research Laboratory, Radboud University Nijmegen Medical Centre, Nijmegen, The Netherlands

AMY VIEIRA, PA-C
Physician Assistant, Department of Orthopedic Surgery, Menlo Medical Clinic, Stanford University Medical Center, Menlo Park, California

J. VOOS, MD
Sports Medicine and Shoulder Service, The Hospital for Special Surgery, New York, New York

I-NING ELAINE WANG, MS
Department of Biomedical Engineering, Biomaterials and Interface Tissue Engineering Laboratory, Columbia University, New York, New York

JAMES WOODALL, Jr., MD
Orthopedic Resident, Department of Orthopedic Surgery, University of Mississippi Medical Center, Jackson, Mississippi

VONDA J. WRIGHT, MD
Stem Cell Research Center, Children's Hospital of Pittsburgh, Rangos Research Center; Department of Orthopaedic Surgery, University of Pittsburgh Medical Center, Pittsburgh, Pennsylvania

Contents

> Skeletal muscle injuries are extremely common, accounting for up to 35%–55% of all sports injuries and quite possibly affecting all musculoskeletal traumas. These injuries result in the formation of fibrosis, which may lead to the development of painful contractures, increases patients' risk for repeat injuries, and limits their ability to return to a baseline or pre-injury level of function. The development of successful therapies for these injuries must consider the pathophysiology of these musculoskeletal conditions. We discuss the direct use of muscle-derived stem cells and some key cell population dynamics as well as the use of clinically applicable modalities that may enhance the local supply of stem cells to the zone of injury by promoting angiogenesis.

> The 4 fibrocartilagenous transition zones of the rotator cuff insertion site are not recreated following surgical repair. Instead, a layer of scar tissue is formed between the tendon and the bone, which makes repairs prone to failure. Growth factors are a group of cytokines that induce mitosis, extracellular matrix production, neovascularization, cell maturation, and differentiation. Research has focused on their ability to augment rotator cuff repairs. Studies have shown that several factors are capable of increasing the strength of repairs in animal models. However, this appears to be accomplished through the production of more scar tissue, as opposed to regeneration of native tissue. It is becoming clear that multiple factors may be needed to regenerate the native tendon-bone insertion site. The optimal timing and vehicle for growth factor delivery have remained elusive. Gene therapy and tissue scaffolds provide promising options for the future, but the engineering still needs to be optimized for clinical use. Growth factor therapy for rotator cuff repairs remains a promising therapeutic for the future; however, much work needs to be done to optimize its effectiveness.

Kai Mithoefer, Timothy R. McAdams, Jason M. Scopp,
and Bert R. Mandelbaum

Articular cartilage injury is observed with increasing frequency in both elite
and amateur athletes and results from the significant joint stress associated particularly with high-impact sports. The lack of spontaneous healing
of these joint surface defects leads to progressive joint pain and mechanical symptoms with resulting functional impairment and limitation of athletic participation. Left untreated, articular cartilage defects can lead to
chronic joint degeneration and athletic disability. Articular cartilage repair
in athletes requires effective and durable joint surface restoration that
can withstand the significant joint stresses generated during athletic activity. Several techniques for articular cartilage repair have been developed
recently, which can successfully restore articular cartilage surfaces and allow for return to high-impact athletics after articular cartilage injury. Besides these existing techniques, new promising scientific concepts and
techniques are emerging that incorporate modern tissue engineering technologies and promise further improvement for the treatment of these challenging injuries in the demanding athletic population.

D. Kendoff, M. Citak, J. Voos, and A.D. Pearle

The use of computer navigation in ACL reconstruction was first established in the mid- 1990s. Initial applications of this new technology focused
on improving the accuracy and repeatability of tunnel placement. More
recent indications focus on intraoperative assessment of knee ligament
dynamic laxity measurements. Computer navigation has been used increasingly as a quantitative measurement tool to assess ACL graft obliquity or visualization of the pivot-shift phenomenon. Applications for PCL
and MCL reconstruction have not been extensively studied thus far,
although specific isometric or laxity measurements could be performed.
Future applications include noninvasive registration techniques to use
navigation as a combined preoperative, intraoperative and postoperative
measurement tool. The purpose of this review is to provide an overview
of the current applications and limitations of navigation in knee ligament
reconstruction by reviewing the currently available literature.

Martha M. Murray

Anterior cruciate ligament (ACL) rupture occurs in hundreds of thousands
of active adolescents and young adults each year. Despite current treatment, posttraumatic osteoarthritis following these injuries is common in
these young patients. Thus, there is widespread clinical and scientific interest in improving patient outcomes and preventing osteoarthritis. The
current emphasis on the removal of the torn ACL and subsequent replacement with a tendon graft (ACL reconstruction) stems from adherence to
a long-held and widely accepted doctrine that the ACL has only a limited
healing response and, therefore, cannot heal or regenerate with suture

repair. Recent work has shown that, despite an active biologic response in the ACL after injury, the two ends of the torn ligament never reconnect. Additional studies have detailed findings after placement of a substitute provisional scaffold in the wound site of the ACL injury to bridge the gap and initiate healing of the ruptured ligament after primary repair. This technique, called enhanced primary repair, has significant potential advantages over current ACL reconstruction techniques, including the preservation of the complex attachment sites and innervation of these structures, thus retaining much of the biomechanical and proprioceptive function of these tissues. This manuscript summarizes the recent in vitro and in vivo studies in the area of enhancing ACL healing using biologic supplementation. Subsequent work in this area may lead to the development of a novel approach to treat this important injury.

Specialized testing procedures allow rehabilitation clinicians and strength and conditioning specialists to measure progress and functional level. Testing will ensure a safe progression throughout the rehabilitative course by providing the needed criteria for advancement. Performance testing quantifies the pure physical nature of athletic performance. Successful rehabilitation can be attained only by following a functional progression. Testing procedures also follow a progression, which begins with basic measures and progresses to functional tests of increasing difficulty that include sports-specific testing before returning to field play. Clinical tests provide both quantitative and qualitative information. These tests not only quantify physiologic response to rehabilitation but also allow the clinician to provide qualitative feedback to an individual during a specific activity. Balance, strength, power, cardiovascular endurance, functional movement, as well as the component of apprehension with sport-specific activity are important and valuable measures in prevention, rehabilitation, and performance programs.

Standardized magnetic resonance imaging (MRI) pulse sequences provide an accurate, reproducible assessment of cartilage morphology. Three-dimensional (3D) modeling techniques enable semiautomated models of the joint surface and thickness measurements, which may eventually prove essential in templating before partial or total joint resurfacing as well as focal cartilage repair. Quantitative MRI techniques, such as T2 mapping, T1 rho, and delayed gadolinium-enhanced MRI of cartilage (dGEMRIC), provide noninvasive information about cartilage and repair tissue biochemistry. Diffusion-weighted imaging (DWI) and diffusion tensor imaging (DTI) demonstrate information regarding the regional anisotropic variation of cartilage ultrastructure. Further research strengthening the association between quantitative MRI and cartilage material properties may predict the functional capacity of native and repaired tissue. MRI provides an essential objective assessment of cartilage regenerative procedures.

The meniscus plays a critical role in load transmission, stability and energy dissipation in the knee joint. Loss of the meniscus leads to joint degeneration and osteoarthritis. An increased understanding of the degenerative changes that occur after meniscectomy made clear that it is beneficial to save as much meniscal tissue as possible. Meniscal repair has become a standard procedure, and partial resection of damaged menisci should be performed as sparingly as possible. However, not all damaged menisci can be treated by partial resection or by repair, making a total meniscectomy inevitable. In these cases, replacement of the resected meniscal tissue by an implant might avoid the articular cartilage degeneration. Different types of meniscal substitutes, such as allografts, collagen, permanent synthetic scaffolds, and biodegradable scaffolds, have been used in experimental and clinical studies. This review highlights the research on these meniscal substitutes and shows that current research is mainly focused on a biological tissue-engineering approach either with or without additional cell-seeding techniques.

Interface tissue engineering is a promising new strategy aimed at the regeneration of tissue interfaces and ultimately enabling the biological fixation of soft tissue grafts used in orthopedic repair and sports medicine. Many ligaments and tendons with direct insertions into subchondral bone exhibit a complex enthesis consisting of several distinct yet continuous regions of soft tissue, noncalcified fibrocartilage, calcified fibrocartilage, and bone. Regeneration of this multi-tissue interface will be critical for functional graft integration and improving long-term clinical outcome. This review highlights current knowledge of the structure–function relationship at the interface, the mechanism of interface regeneration, and the strategic biomimicry implemented in stratified scaffold design for interface tissue engineering and multi-tissue regeneration. Potential challenges and future directions in this emerging field are also discussed. It is anticipated that interface tissue engineering will lead to the design of a new generation of integrative fixation devices for soft tissue repair, and it will be instrumental for the development of integrated musculoskeletal tissue systems with biomimetic complexity and functionality.

FORTHCOMING ISSUES

RECENT ISSUES

THE CLINICS ARE NOW AVAILABLE ONLINE!

Access your subscription at:
www.theclinics.com

Foreword

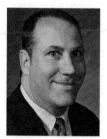

Mark D. Miller, MD
Consulting Editor

The media keeps hyping all of the new and exhilarating advances in orthopedics, but it certainly takes some time for them to make it into our operating rooms. There is a lot of exciting and ongoing research on stem cells, growth factors, imaging, computer navigation, tissue engineering, and articular cartilage repair—but where do we stand and what (and when!) is the future? I asked Dr. Scott Rodeo, who is at the forefront of many of these developments, to play Buck Rogers for this issue and give us a glimpse into the future.

Dr. Rodeo has done an excellent job of bringing together the new generation of experts to give us some insight. This issue covers all of the areas that I mentioned above—and more! There are a lot of cool advances right around the corner... really! So read on and let's set a course for our future!

Mark D. Miller, MD
Department of Orthopaedic Surgery
Division of Sports Medicine
University of Virginia Health System
P.O. Box 800753
UVA Dept of Orthopaedic Surgery
Charlottesville, VA 22908-0159, USA

E-mail address:
mdm3p@virginia.edu (M.D. Miller)

Clin Sports Med 28 (2009) xiii
doi:10.1016/j.csm.2008.10.001
0278-5919/08/$ – see front matter © 2008 Elsevier Inc. All rights reserved.

sportsmed.theclinics.com

Preface

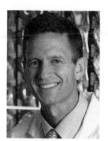

Scott A. Rodeo, MD
Guest Editor

This issue of *Clinics in Sports Medicine* explores a number of novel diagnostic modalities and treatment techniques for musculoskeletal injuries and diseases. Progress in diagnosis and treatment in all areas of medicine are dependent upon basic and clinical research. Advances in numerous areas have improved our understanding of the basic biology of tissue degeneration and healing. New information in areas such as stem cell biology, genetic modification of cells, cell signalling, mechanotransduction, cytokine function, and developmental biology hold tremendous potential for application to the repair and regeneration of ligament, tendon, meniscus, and articular cartilage.

In this issue of *Clinics in Sports Medicine*, leading experts have written summaries of the current state of the art in areas related to articular cartilage imaging, allograft tissue transplantation, the use of growth factors in healing, tissue engineering, concussion management, and rehabilitation. These reviews summarize emerging treatment options and highlight areas for further research. Our job as clinicians is to critically evaluate these new ideas and then begin to incorporate them into our daily practices. The information presented here will also help to define research agendas and stimulate avenues for further research. It is my hope that you, the reader, will find something of interest that will apply to your current practice as well as stimulate new ideas that will lead to future progress.

Scott A. Rodeo, MD
The Hospital for Special Surgery
535 East 70th Street
New York, NY 10021

E-mail address:
rodeos@hss.edu (S.A. Rodeo)

Clin Sports Med 28 (2009) xv
doi:10.1016/j.csm.2008.08.001
0278-5919/08/$ – see front matter © 2008 Elsevier Inc. All rights reserved.

Stem Cells for the Treatment of Skeletal Muscle Injury

Andres J. Quintero, MD[a,b,c,d], Vonda J. Wright, MD[a,e], Freddie H. Fu, MD[f],
Johnny Huard, PhD[a,b,c,d],*

KEYWORDS

- Sports injury • Stem cells • Tissue engineering • Fibrosis
- Regeneration • Skeletal muscle

Skeletal muscle injury can result form a variety of mechanisms, including contusion, strain, laceration, or a combination of these mechanisms.[1–5] It is also possible for skeletal muscle injury to result from indirect sequelae of overexertion or direct injury, such as through ischemia and neurologic impairment secondary to exercise-induced or traumatic compartment syndromes.[6–15] These injuries are extremely common, accounting for up to 35%–55% of all sports injuries and quite possibly affecting all musculoskeletal traumas.[16–18] The associated morbidity is considerable, as these injuries portend professional and recreational athletes to developing painful contractures and muscle atrophy, requiring prolonged recovery periods, increasing the risk for recurrent injury, and in some cases, limiting patients' abilities to return to baseline or pre-injury levels of activity.[1,6,19] Significant efforts are being made to improve the current treatment of skeletal muscle trauma.

Currently, the treatment of these injuries by and large consists of rest, ice, compression, and elevation (RICE), although other advocated treatments include the local application of heat, immobilization, and passive range of motion exercises as well as non-steroidal anti-inflammatory drugs (NSAIDs), intramuscular corticosteroids, and even surgery.[1–4] In many instances, however, these therapies remain suboptimal.

[a] Stem Cell Research Center, Children's Hospital of Pittsburgh, 4100 Rangos Research Center, 3640 Fifth Avenue, Pittsburgh, PA 15213-2582, USA
[b] Department of Orthopaedic Surgery, University of Pittsburgh Medical Center, Pittsburgh, PA 15213, USA
[c] Department of Microbiology and Molecular Genetics, E1240 BST, 200 Lothrop Street, Pittsburgh, PA 15261, USA
[d] Department of Bioengineering, University of Pittsburgh, 749 Benedum Hall, PA 15261, USA
[e] Department of Orthopaedic Surgery, University of Pittsburgh Medical Center, 3200 South West Street, Pittsburgh, PA 15203, USA
[f] Department of Orthopaedic Surgery, University of Pittsburgh Medical Center, 3471 5th Avenue, Suite 1010, Pittsburgh, PA 15213, USA
* Corresponding author. University of Pittsburgh School of Medicine, Children's Hospital of Pittsburgh, 4100 Rangos Research Center, 3640 Fifth Avenue, Pittsburgh, PA 15213-2582.
E-mail address: jhuard@pitt.edu (J. Huard).

Clin Sports Med 28 (2009) 1–11
doi:10.1016/j.csm.2008.08.009
0278-5919/08/$ – see front matter. Published by Elsevier Inc.

sportsmed.theclinics.com

During the past decade, there have been sophisticated advances in rehabilitation, biomechanics, cell therapies, and tissue engineering with the goal of enhancing current therapies. As research in cell therapy and tissue engineering has progressed, it is clear that successful therapies must be based on an understanding of the basic pathophysiology of skeletal muscle injury.

PATHOPHYSIOLOGY OF SKELETAL MUSCLE INJURY

The pathophysiology of skeletal muscle injury is characterized by a sequence of events consisting of degeneration, inflammation, myofiber regeneration, and the formation of fibrotic scar tissue, as described below in detail and illustrated in **Fig. 1**.

Degeneration and Inflammation

Immediately following injury, there is a phase of myofiber degeneration, which is initiated by the release of proteases into the tissue stroma; these proteases autodigest myofibers and thereby, release tissue debris along the zone of injury.[20] Within the time frame that this occurs, there is a chemotaxis of neutrophils and macrophages to this area, at which point the local debris is phagocytosed and processed by macrophages to induce a local inflammatory response.[21–24] Although it appears that macrophages may in part be a culprit by initiating an inflammatory response, some studies indicate that these cells also secrete various growth factors that directly contribute to tissue regeneration. Additionally, macrophages stimulate the paracrine release of cytokines and other chemotactic factors by T cells, which may locally recruit progenitor and satellite cells with the capacity for muscle regeneration.[25–31] Some of the critical cytokines that orchestrate this local response include interleukin [IL]-1, -6, and -8 as well as insulin growth factor [IGF]-1. It is clear from this initial sequence of events, then, that the inflammatory response may be conducive to the repair of skeletal muscle after injury. In the event that this event is blunted, such as through the use of NSAIDs or intramuscular corticosteroid injections, the tangible clinical benefits of blunting the classic inflammatory symptoms of pain (dolor), heat (calor), erythema (rubor), and swelling (tumor) must be weighed against the cost of potentially delaying and reducing the extent of tissue healing that may be mediated by infiltrating progenitor cells. Some evidence from animal studies suggests that the blocking the

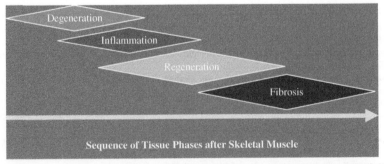

Fig.1. Skeletal muscle injury pathology. After injury, there is a degeneration phase followed by inflammation. This inflammatory response locally recruits progenitor cells to the zone of injury for muscle repair. The reparative phase can last up to 3 wk and is followed by a deleterious rise of TGF-B that induces fibrosis, which places patients at increased risk for recurrent injury, developing painful contractures and requiring lengthy recovery periods from which there is often an incomplete return to baseline function.

cyclooxygenase-2 pathway with prostaglandin inhibitors such as NSAIDs compromises the histologic quality of muscle repair and may even result in a functional compromise.[32,33] This may in large part result, from the upregulation of transforming growth factor [TGF]-β1, which inhibits myogenic precursor cells and augments fibrosis.[34]

Regeneration

The subsequent phase of myofiber regeneration may begin as early as 24 hours following injury, as evidenced by the cytokine-mediated induction of local satellite cells which previously lay dormant between the basal lamina and sarcolemma; it is not until at least 3 to 5 days after injury, however, that the complete formation of new, centronucleated myofibers can be detected histologically.[7,27,35]

It is likely that a crucial event in the regeneration phase is the differentiation of satellite cells into myotubules and myofibers. To date, these progenitor cells are perhaps the best characterized and are often referred to as "muscle stem cells" given their predilection to the myogenic lineage. There are, however, other populations isolated from skeletal muscle, including muscle side-population cells, mesoangioblasts, pericytes, and postnatal muscle-derived stem cells (MDSCs), which appear to be multipotent.[36–42]

Although the origin and relationship of these additional progenitor cells to muscle stem cells remain to be fully elucidated, emerging evidence suggests that MDSCs represent a highly purified and unique population of stem cells that have several advantages for regenerative medicine over other populations. These advantages by and large consist of their longer-term survival after implantation into skeletal muscle compared with myoblasts; their remarkable multi-potency (**Fig. 2**) and their potential for

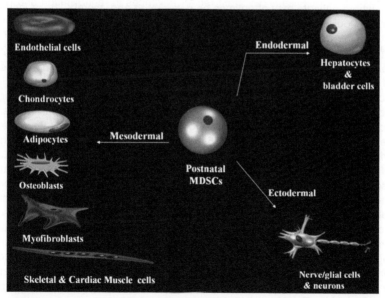

Fig. 2. Multipotency of muscle-derived stem cells, the authors' laboratory has previously isolated muscle-derived stem cells from mice. These cells are remarkably pluripotent and can undergo long-term expansion. Accordingly, MDSCs are ideal for regenerative medicine.

long-term regeneration, with up to 300 population doublings (PDs) before becoming senescent compared with population doublings of 130 to 250 for embryonic stem cells.[37,40,43–46] Additionally, MDSCs can be efficiently transduced with antifibrotic and regenerative factors that may enhance skeletal muscle healing.[44,47,48]

Since the discovery of MDSCs, a topic of interest has been their origin. As of recently, there is convincing evidence that these cells are likely derived from the vascular endothelium.[49,50] Accordingly, a growing focus in research on skeletal muscle repair has not only involved finding ways to use MDSCs for repairing the zone of injury but also to augment the local vascular supply as a way to provide a steady source of MDSCs.[42,44,50–52]

Fibrosis

Perhaps the greatest limitation for patients that results from the pathophysiology of skeletal muscle injury is the formation of dense fibrotic scar tissue. It is clear that fibrosis is induced by a deleterious rise in the cytokine transforming growth factor (TGF)-B1 after injury.[46] In the presence of this cytokine, MDSCs and other myogenic cells differentiate into myofibroblasts that produce collagen type I, the major component of fibrotic tissue.[8,34,45,53] Ultimately, fibrosis can prevent patients from returning to their baseline function, in part by preventing the formation of new axons toward myofibers and contributes to a decline in muscle contractility and range of motion.[54,55] The pain that results from fibrosis is also a limiting factor in the recovery of patients during both rehabilitation and in the long-term.

Although not currently used clinically in this capacity, several agents that block TGF-B1 have proven to be remarkably antifibrotic, including gamma-interferon, suramin, and decorin.[56–58] Fortunately, the commercially available diuretic, losartan, has also been shown to have a significant antifibrotic effect along the zone of skeletal muscle injury in Sprague Dawley rats.[59] Although clinical trials with this medication are feasible, they must be used with caution in settings of musculoskeletal traumas and athletic injuries, where patients may oftentimes be dehydrated and, thereby, be at increased risk for developing acute renal insufficiency.

Skeletal Muscle Engineering with Muscle-Derived Stem Cells

The transplantation of stem cells into aberrant or injured tissue has long been a central goal of regenerative medicine and tissue engineering. This translation of basic science research on muscle repair with autologous MDSCs to the bedside has been spearheaded by preliminary trials to treat stress urinary incontinence. One trial has resulted in successful cases over a 1-year period following the implantation of these cells to restore detrusor muscle function, with 5 out of 8 females reporting improvements, 1 achieving complete continence, and none sustaining any adverse outcomes.[60] Larger clinical trials using MDSCs to treat this disease entity are planned for the near future.

Presently, most reports on research using stem cell therapies for muscle regeneration are limited to animal models. Successful results have been reported for Duchene Muscular Dystrophy models, in which dystrophin can be restored following the systemic delivery of various stem cells.[40,61,62] Perhaps more relevant to sports injuries, Kinnaird and colleagues[63] developed an ischemic model in which Balb/C mice underwent ligation of the femoral artery; compared with controls, mice that later received distal injections of marrow-derived stromal cells on the affected limb displayed significantly better perfusion and appearance, had a lower incidence of autoamputation, and developed less fibrosis and atrophy.

Although perhaps a more severe form of ischemia, this ischemic model may translate in part to the ischemia that may occur from an exercise-induced compartment syndrome, raising the possibility that the local injection of autologous stem cells early during the development of limb ischemia from such a mechanism is worthy of further investigation. Presently, although the authors' laboratory is investigating the role of directly implanted MDSCs into contused skeletal muscle following contusion, the benefits of doing so have not been determined. It is hoped that reports on this will follow in the near future.

Although the literature may often refer to MDSCs as a homogeneous population, these stem cells are quite heterogeneous, differing in how efficiently different populations regenerate skeletal muscle in vivo. Research on sex-related differences in the regeneration of skeletal muscle for Duchenne muscular dystrophy models shows that, regardless of the host's sex, female MDCSs are significantly superior to male MDSCs in regenerating and repairing skeletal muscle.[52] The use of MDSCs to repair bone and cartilage is also influenced by the gender of the cells and the host animals, with the male MDSCs displaying a superior regeneration index than their female counterpart.[64,65] This may in large part be due to different embryonic developmental patterns that occur in female and male embryogenesis. Deasy and colleagues[66,67] also found that in skeletal muscle experiments where donor MDSCs are sex-matched, female hosts are also superior, a finding that is supported by other studies suggesting that the hormonal milieu of the female host skeletal muscle is better suited for donor cell transplantation. The role of immune rejection does not appear to explain the lower regeneration index of male donor cells transplanted into female hosts, because these sex differences were also identified when using severe combined immunodeficient host mice. This confirms that these sex differences may indeed occur because females are superior donors and hosts for MDSC-mediated skeletal muscle regeneration. Although further studies are necessary to show a similar phenomenon with human cells, future therapeutic advances in skeletal muscle healing with MDSCs can greatly benefit from these important gender differences observed with MDSC.

Skeletal Muscle Engineering with Angiogenic Modalities: Exercise and Neuromuscular Electrical Stimulation

Aside from directly implanting stem cells into skeletal muscle, significant attention now focuses on promoting angiogenesis to activate resident satellite cells and provide a long-lasting portal through which MDSCs can derive, ultimately to aid in skeletal muscle healing. With clear evidence that exercise promotes cardiac and skeletal muscle perfusion, several studies now show this is because muscle contraction, such as through voluntary exercise or neuromuscular electrical stimulation (NMES), induces the formation of new vessels and the expansion of existing vascular trees.[68–70]

Aside from promoting angiogenesis, several other mechanisms exist through which exercise can enhance healing. For instance, exercise increases the serum concentrations of matrix metalloproteinases (MMPs), which directly digest fibrotic scar tissue, regulate the secretion of pro-regenerative growth factors such as insulin-like growth factor, and may also mobilize stem cells.[71–74] Moreover, several studies show that exercise-induced hypoxia promoted skeletal muscle healing by elevating the circulating concentrations of hypoxia-induced factor, stromal-cell derived factor, and erythropoietin, each of which mobilizes endothelial progenitor stem cells from the bone marrow to coordinate the neovascularization of hypoxic tissues.[75–82] In light of this information, there is certainly potential for combining MMPs and stem cells for direct implantation as well as MMPs with conservative means of promoting angiogenesis, such as voluntary exercise and, as will be discussed below, NMES.

Based on this information, it is possible that, at least for some instances of skeletal muscle injury, the more traditional therapy of rest may jeopardize an opportunity to locally recruit stem cells to the zone of injury. It is also possible that through controlled and monitored exercise regimens in appropriately selected patients, perhaps initiated before the completion or the regeneration phase of skeletal muscle injury, the activation and infiltration of stem cells to the zone of injury may increase and enhance regeneration. Further studies may be necessary to determine whether rest is deleterious to healing after injury, whether certain exercises are safe and clinically beneficial, and, if so, whether the timing of exercise rehabilitation relative to the onset of injury influences outcomes.

As with exercise, another modality that appears to promote angiogenesis and skeletal muscle healing after injury is NMES. Although the data linking stem cell activation and recruitment to NMES are lacking, there is evidence that this modality promotes angiogenesis.[70,83] As with exercise, it appears that tissue hypoxia induced during NMES may play a role in promoting angiogenesis, although the exact mechanism requires further elucidation.[84] It has been demonstrated in the authors' laboratory that among 9-week old male C57BL/10J mice, prophylactic and post-injury NMES significantly enhances the percent capillary area of the tibialis anterior (unpublished data.) Additionally, at 5 and 10 days after injury, the percentage regeneration significantly increases, and the percentage fibrosis significantly decreases along the zone of injury in mice undergoing prophylactic electrical stimulation 3 times weekly for 2 weeks (unpublished data.) Among mice undergoing post-injury NMES, we had the same findings for fibrosis, but were only able to detect a significant increase in the percentage regeneration at 10 days after injury (unpublished data).

One reason why prophylactic NMES may be superior to post-injury stimulation is that by promoting angiogenesis early on, the regenerative phase of skeletal muscle injury will begin to occur in the presence of more MDSCs derived from the vascular endothelium and more infiltrating growth factors that activate dormant satellite cells. With post-injury stimulation, these cells and factors may come into the zone of injury beyond the optimal time window for tissue repair. Although speculative at the present time, this would be consistent with proposition above that early exercise rehabilitation programs may be beneficial in some cases of skeletal muscle injury, although clinical studies are necessary to support this. This may also be similar to the process of fracture repair, in which relatively early fracture stabilization is oftentimes necessary to prevent the progression to fracture non-union.[85] Therefore, more studies are required to better delineate the temporal relationship of skeletal muscle injury, NMES, and other therapeutic interventions, such as the implantation of stem cells directly into the zone of injury to optimize skeletal muscle healing responses.

SUMMARY

Among the most commonly prescribed treatments for skeletal muscle injuries are rest, ice application, compression, and elevation as well as heat application and either immobilization or passive range of motion exercises. In many instances, however, these therapies remain suboptimal.

Based on current knowledge, the inflammatory response that follows injury promotes skeletal muscle regeneration, perhaps in part by locally recruiting stem cells through chemotaxis to the zone of injury. Although the therapeutic administration of steroids and NSAIDs may provide symptomatic relief by combating inflammation, there is evidence that this blunts the regenerative response and may actually promote fibrosis.

Current research has linked angiogenesis to skeletal muscle healing and indicates that blood vessels are probably the origin of MDSCs. Because voluntary exercise and NMES promote angiogenesis, it is possible that in appropriately selected patients, a feasible therapeutic alternative to rest and immobilization for skeletal muscle injury may consist of controlled and monitored exercise programs as well as NMES. Future studies may need to determine whether rest is deleterious to skeletal muscle healing and which exercises are safe and clinically efficacious for various patterns and locations of injury. Similarly, a feasible alternative to current pharmacologic therapies may include losartan, although the use of this medication for treating skeletal muscle injury is not currently approved by the United States Food and Drug Administration.

In light of recent successful clinical trials on the direct implantation of MDSCs to treat urinary incontinence secondary to detrusor muscle dysfunction, the future of stem cell therapy for skeletal muscle injury may be closer than ever to translation into clinical studies. Such studies must continue to characterize and make use of the optimal MDSC populations as well as examine MDSC transplantation in combination with pro-regenerative and antifibrotic agents such as MMPs and losartan.

REFERENCES

1. Lehto MU, Jarvinen MJ. Muscle injuries, their healing process and treatment. Ann Chir Gynaecol 1991;80(2):102–8.
2. Levine WN, Bergfeld JA, Tessendorf W, et al. Intramuscular corticosteroid injection for hamstring injuries. A 13-year experience in the National Football League. Am J Sports Med 2000;28(3):297–300.
3. Jarvinen MJ, Lehto MU. The effects of early mobilisation and immobilisation on the healing process following muscle injuries. Sports Med 1993;15(2):78–89.
4. Hurme T, Kalimo H, Lehto M, et al. Healing of skeletal muscle injury: an ultrastructural and immunohistochemical study. Med Sci Sports Exerc 1991;23(7):801–10.
5. Jarvinen TA, Jarvinen TL, Kaariainen M, et al. Muscle injuries: biology and treatment. Am J Sports Med 2005;33(5):745–64.
6. Huard J, Li Y, Fu FH. Muscle injuries and repair: current trends in research. J Bone Joint Surg Am 2002;84(5):822–32.
7. Li YCJ, Huard J. Muscle injury and repair. Curr Opin Orthop 2001;12:409–15.
8. Cetinus E, Uzel M, Bilgic E, et al. Exercise induced compartment syndrome in a professional footballer. Br J Sports Med 2004;38(2):227–9.
9. Edmundsson D, Toolanen G, Sojka P. Chronic compartment syndrome also affects nonathletic subjects: a prospective study of 63 cases with exercise-induced lower leg pain. Acta Orthop 2007;78(1):136–42.
10. Howard JL, Mohtadi NG, Wiley JP. Evaluation of outcomes in patients following surgical treatment of chronic exertional compartment syndrome in the leg. Clin J Sport Med 2000;10(3):176–84.
11. Leppilahti J, Tervonen O, Herva R, et al. Acute bilateral exercise-induced medial compartment syndrome of the thigh. Correlation of repeated MRI with clinicopathological findings. Int J Sports Med 2002;23(8):610–5.
12. Levine WN. Exercise-induced compartment syndrome. Am J Knee Surg 1995; 8(4):119.
13. Litwiller DV, Amrami KK, Dahm DL, et al. Chronic exertional compartment syndrome of the lower extremities: improved screening using a novel dual birdcage coil and in-scanner exercise protocol. Skeletal Radiol 2007;36(11):1067–75.
14. Robinson MS, Parekh AA, Smith WR, et al. Bilateral exercise induced exertional compartment syndrome resulting in acute compartment loss: a case report. J Trauma 2008;65(1):225–7.

15. Schissel DJ, Godwin J. Effort-related chronic compartment syndrome of the lower extremity. Mil Med 1999;164(11):830–2.
16. Dyson R, Buchanan M, Hale T. Incidence of sports injuries in elite competitive and recreational windsurfers. Br J Sports Med 2006;40(4):346–50.
17. Stevenson MR, Hamer P, Finch CF, et al. Sport, age, and sex specific incidence of sports injuries in Western Australia. Br J Sports Med 2000;34(3):188–94.
18. Brooks JH, Fuller CW, Kemp SP, et al. Incidence, risk, and prevention of hamstring muscle injuries in professional rugby union. Am J Sports Med 2006;34(8):1297–306.
19. Garrett WE Jr. Muscle strain injuries: clinical and basic aspects. Med Sci Sports Exerc 1990;22(4):436–43.
20. Mbebi C, Hantai D, Jandrot-Perrus M, et al. Protease nexin I expression is up-regulated in human skeletal muscle by injury-related factors. J Cell Physiol 1999;179(3):305–14.
21. Orimo S, Hiyamuta E, Arahata K, et al. Analysis of inflammatory cells and complement C3 in bupivacaine-induced myonecrosis. Muscle Nervo 1991; 14(6):515–20.
22. Tidball JG, Berchenko E, Frenette J. Macrophage invasion does not contribute to muscle membrane injury during inflammation. J Leukoc Biol 1999;65(4):492–8.
23. Warren GL, Hulderman T, Jensen N, et al. Physiological role of tumor necrosis factor alpha in traumatic muscle injury. FASEB J 2002;16(12):1630–2.
24. Mitchell CA, McGeachie JK, Grounds MD. Cellular differences in the regeneration of murine skeletal muscle: a quantitative histological study in SJL/J and BALB/c mice. Cell Tissue Res 1992;269(1):159–66.
25. Tidball JG. Inflammatory processes in muscle injury and repair. Am J Physiol Regul Integr Comp Physiol 2005;288(2):R345–53.
26. Cantini M, Carraro U. Macrophage-released factor stimulates selectively myogenic cells in primary muscle culture. J Neuropathol Exp Neurol 1995;54(1):121–8.
27. Hurme T, Kalimo H. Activation of myogenic precursor cells after muscle injury. Med Sci Sports Exerc 1992;24(2):197–205.
28. Massimino ML, Rapizzi E, Cantini M, et al. ED2+ macrophages increase selectively myoblast proliferation in muscle cultures. Biochem Biophys Res Commun 1997;235(3):754–9.
29. Robertson TA, Maley MA, Grounds MD, et al. The role of macrophages in skeletal muscle regeneration with particular reference to chemotaxis. Exp Cell Res 1993;207(2):321–31.
30. DiPietro LA. Wound healing: the role of the macrophage and other immune cells. Shock 1995;4(4):233–40.
31. Summan M, Warren GL, Mercer RR, et al. Macrophages and skeletal muscle regeneration: a clodronate-containing liposome depletion study. Am J Physiol Regul Integr Comp Physiol 2006;290(6):R1488–95.
32. Shen W, Prisk V, Li Y, et al. Inhibited skeletal muscle healing in cyclooxygenase-2 gene-deficient mice: the role of PGE2 and PGF2alpha. J Appl Physiol 2006; 101(4):1215–21.
33. Mishra DK, Friden J, Schmitz MC, et al. Anti-inflammatory medication after muscle injury. A treatment resulting in short-term improvement but subsequent loss of muscle function. J Bone Joint Surg Am 1995;77(10):1510–9.
34. Shen W, Li Y, Tang Y, et al. NS-398, a cyclooxygenase-2-specific inhibitor, delays skeletal muscle healing by decreasing regeneration and promoting fibrosis. Am J Pathol 2005;167(4):1105–17.

35. Rantanen J, Hurme T, Lukka R, et al. Satellite cell proliferation and the expression of myogenin and desmin in regenerating skeletal muscle: evidence for two different populations of satellite cells. Lab Invest 1995;72(3):341–7.
36. Peault B, Rudnicki M, Torrente Y, et al. Stem and progenitor cells in skeletal muscle development, maintenance, and therapy. Mol Ther 2007;15(5):867–77.
37. Lee JY, Qu-Petersen Z, Cao B, et al. Clonal isolation of muscle-derived cells capable of enhancing muscle regeneration and bone healing. J Cell Biol 2000; 150(5):1085–100.
38. Asakura A, Komaki M, Rudnicki M. Muscle satellite cells are multipotential stem cells that exhibit myogenic, osteogenic, and adipogenic differentiation. Differentiation 2001;68(4–5):245–53.
39. Wada MR, Inagawa-Ogashiwa M, Shimizu S, et al. Generation of different fates from multipotent muscle stem cells. Development 2002;129(12):2987–95.
40. Cao B, Zheng B, Jankowski RJ, et al. Muscle stem cells differentiate into haematopoietic lineages but retain myogenic potential. Nat Cell Biol 2003;5(7):640–6.
41. Musgrave DS, Fu FH, Huard J. Gene therapy and tissue engineering in orthopaedic surgery. J Am Acad Orthop Surg 2002;10(1):6–15.
42. Peng H, Huard J. Muscle-derived stem cells for musculoskeletal tissue regeneration and repair. Transpl Immunol 2004;12(3-4):311–9.
43. Deasy BM, Gharaibeh BM, Pollett JB, et al. Long-term self-renewal of postnatal muscle-derived stem cells. Mol Biol Cell 2005;16(7):3323–33.
44. Qu-Petersen Z, Deasy B, Jankowski R, et al. Identification of a novel population of muscle stem cells in mice: potential for muscle regeneration. J Cell Biol 2002; 157(5):851–64.
45. Li Y, Huard J. Differentiation of muscle-derived cells into myofibroblasts in injured skeletal muscle. Am J Pathol 2002;161(3):895–907.
46. Li Y, Foster W, Deasy BM, et al. Transforming growth factor-beta1 induces the differentiation of myogenic cells into fibrotic cells in injured skeletal muscle: a key event in muscle fibrogenesis. Am J Pathol 2004;164(3):1007–19.
47. Irintchev A, Wernig A. Muscle damage and repair in voluntarily running mice: strain and muscle differences. Cell Tissue Res 1987;249(3):509–21.
48. Qu Z, Balkir L, van Deutekom JC, et al. Development of approaches to improve cell survival in myoblast transfer therapy. J Cell Biol 1998;142(5):1257–67.
49. Tavian M, Zheng B, Oberlin E, et al. The vascular wall as a source of stem cells. Ann N Y Acad Sci 2005;1044:41–50.
50. Zheng B, Cao B, Crisan M, et al. Prospective identification of myogenic endothelial cells in human skeletal muscle. Nat Biotechnol 2007;25(9):1025–34.
51. Deasy BM, Li Y, Huard J. Tissue engineering with muscle-derived stem cells. Curr Opin Biotechnol 2004;15(5):419–23.
52. Deasy BM, Lu A, Tebbets JC, et al. A role for cell sex in stem cell-mediated skeletal muscle regeneration: female cells have higher muscle regeneration efficiency. J Cell Biol 2007;177(1):73–86.
53. Ghosh AK. Factors involved in the regulation of type I collagen gene expression: implication in fibrosis. Exp Biol Med (Maywood) 2002;227(5):301–14.
54. Kaariainen M, Jarvinen T, Jarvinen M, et al. Relation between myofibers and connective tissue during muscle injury repair. Scand J Med Sci Sports 2000;10(6): 332–7.
55. Shanmugasundaram TK. Post-injection fibrosis of skeletal muscle: a clinical problem. A personal series of 169 cases. Int Orthop 1980;4(1):31–7.
56. Foster W, Li Y, Usas A, et al. Gamma interferon as an antifibrosis agent in skeletal muscle. J Orthop Res 2003;21(5):798–804.

57. Fukushima K, Badlani N, Usas A, et al. The use of an antifibrosis agent to improve muscle recovery after laceration. Am J Sports Med 2001;29(4):394–402.
58. Kloen P, Jennings CL, Gebhardt MC, et al. Suramin inhibits growth and transforming growth factor-beta 1 (TGF-beta 1) binding in osteosarcoma cell lines. Eur J Cancer 1994;30A(5):678–82.
59. Bedair HS, Karthikeyan T, Quintero AJ, et al. Angiotensin II receptor blockade administered after injury improves muscle regeneration and decreases fibrosis in normal skeletal muscle. Am J Sports Med 2008;36(8):1548–55.
60. Carr LK, Steele D, Steele S, et al. 1-year follow-up of autologous muscle-derived stem cell injection pilot study to treat stress urinary incontinence. Int Urogynecol J Pelvic Floor Dysfunct 2008;58.
61. Torrente Y, Tremblay JP, Pisati F, et al. Intraarterial injection of muscle-derived CD34(+)Sca-1(+) stem cells restores dystrophin in mdx mice. J Cell Biol 2001; 152(2):335–48.
62. Bachrach E, Perez AI, Choi YH, et al. Muscle engraftment of myogenic progenitor cells following intraarterial transplantation. Muscle Nerve 2006;34(1):44–52.
63. Kinnaird T, Stabile E, Burnett MS, et al. Local delivery of marrow-derived stromal cells augments collateral perfusion through paracrine mechanisms. Circulation 2004;109(12):1543–9.
64. Corsi KA, Pollett JB, Phillippi JA, et al. Osteogenic potential of postnatal skeletal muscle-derived stem cells is influenced by donor sex. J Bone Miner Res 2007; 22(10):1592–602.
65. Matsumoto TKS, Meszaros LB, Corsi KA, et al. Potential of muscle-derived stem cells: implication for cartilage regeneration & repair. Arthritis Rheum, in press.
66. Steinlein P, Wessely O, Meyer S, et al. Primary, self-renewing erythroid progenitors develop through activation of both tyrosine kinase and steroid hormone receptors. Curr Biol 1995;5(2):191–204.
67. Jilka RL, Hangoc G, Girasole G, et al. Increased osteoclast development after estrogen loss: mediation by interleukin-6. Science 1992;257(5066):88–91.
68. Bellafiore M, Sivverini G, Palumbo D, et al. Increased cx43 and angiogenesis in exercised mouse hearts. Int J Sports Med 2007;28(9):749–55.
69. Efthimiadou A, Asimakopoulos B, Nikolettos N, et al. The angiogenetic effect of intramuscular administration of b-FGF and a-FGF on cardiac muscle: the influence of exercise on muscle angiogenesis. J Sports Sci 2006;24(8):849–54.
70. Ljubicic V, Adhihetty PJ, Hood DA. Application of animal models: chronic electrical stimulation-induced contractile activity. Can J Appl Physiol 2005;30(5): 625–43.
71. Suhr F, Brixius K, de Marees M, et al. Effects of short-term vibration and hypoxia during high-intensity cycling exercise on circulating levels of angiogenic regulators in humans. J Appl Physiol 2007;103(2):474–83.
72. Bedair H, Liu TT, Kaar JL, et al. Matrix metalloproteinase-1 therapy improves muscle healing. J Appl Physiol 2007;102(6):2338–45.
73. Fowlkes JL, Serra DM, Nagase H, et al. MMPs are IGFBP-degrading proteinases: implications for cell proliferation and tissue growth. Ann N Y Acad Sci 1999;878: 696–9.
74. Fowlkes JL, Serra DM, Bunn RC, et al. Regulation of insulin-like growth factor (IGF)-I action by matrix metalloproteinase-3 involves selective disruption of IGF-I/IGF-binding protein-3 complexes. Endocrinology 2004;145(2):620–6.
75. Tepper OM, Capla JM, Galiano RD, et al. Adult vasculogenesis occurs through in situ recruitment, proliferation, and tubulization of circulating bone marrow-derived cells. Blood 2005;105(3):1068–77.

76. Heissig B, Hattori K, Dias S, et al. Recruitment of stem and progenitor cells from the bone marrow niche requires MMP-9 mediated release of kit-ligand. Cell 2002; 109(5):625–37.
77. Ceradini DJ, Kulkarni AR, Callaghan MJ, et al. Progenitor cell trafficking is regulated by hypoxic gradients through HIF-1 induction of SDF-1. Nat Med 2004; 10(8):858–64.
78. Fandrey J. Oxygen-dependent and tissue-specific regulation of erythropoietin gene expression. Am J Physiol Regul Integr Comp Physiol 2004;286(6):R977–88.
79. Forsythe JA, Jiang BH, Iyer NV, et al. Activation of vascular endothelial growth factor gene transcription by hypoxia-inducible factor 1. Mol Cell Biol 1996; 16(9):4604–13.
80. Jelkmann W. Biology of erythropoietin. Clin Investig 1994;72(6 Suppl):S3–10.
81. Bahlmann FH, De Groot K, Spandau JM, et al. Erythropoietin regulates endothelial progenitor cells. Blood 2004;103(3):921–6.
82. Bahlmann FH, DeGroot K, Duckert T, et al. Endothelial progenitor cell proliferation and differentiation is regulated by erythropoietin. Kidney Int 2003;64(5):1648–52.
83. Nagasaka M, Kohzuki M, Fujii T, et al. Effect of low-voltage electrical stimulation on angiogenic growth factors in ischaemic rat skeletal muscle. Clin Exp Pharmacol Physiol 2006;33(7):623–7.
84. Hudlicka O, Milkiewicz M, Cotter MA, et al. Hypoxia and expression of VEGF-A protein in relation to capillary growth in electrically stimulated rat and rabbit skeletal muscles. Exp Physiol 2002;87(3):373–81.
85. Sumner-Smith G. Delayed unions and nonunions. Diagnosis, pathophysiology, and treatment. Vet Clin North Am Small Anim Pract 1991;21(4):745–60.

Growth Factors for Rotator Cuff Repair

Lawrence V. Gulotta, MD, Scott A. Rodeo, MD*

KEYWORDS

- Tendon biology • Cytokines • BMP • Growth factors
- Gene therapy • Repair scaffolds

Rotator cuff repair surgeries are one of the most common procedures performed by orthopedic surgeons, with over 250,000 performed annually in the United States alone. Despite its prevalence, there is concern regarding the ability of the rotator cuff to heal back to the insertion site on the humerus following repair. Clinical studies have shown radiographic failures at the repair site at 2 years in anywhere from 11% to 95% of patients, depending on the size and chronicity of the tear, presence of fatty infiltration, and the age and general health status of the patient.[1–6] Although patients with re-tears or failed healing may have pain relief, these studies show that they have inferior functional results when compared with patients with healed repairs.[2,3] An understanding of the histology and biology that occur during the healing process may lead to therapies that can improve the healing rate and improve the functional results of patients following repair.

Our understanding of tendon healing is largely based on animal studies because there is little histologic information on healing rotator cuff tendons in human beings. From this animal data, it is known that rotator cuff healing occurs in 3 stages: inflammation, repair, and remodeling (**Fig. 1**).[7] In the inflammatory stage, inflammatory cells migrate into the repair site guided by chemotactic factors followed by an influx of blood vessels and fibroblasts. In the repair phase, several growth factors are upregulated that induce cellular proliferation and matrix deposition. Finally, this tissue undergoes remodeling due to extracellular matrix turnover mediated by matrix metalloproteinases (MMPs).

At the conclusion of the healing process, a normal rotator cuff insertion site is not regenerated. Normally, the rotator cuff inserts into bone through 4 distinct transition zones: tendon, unmineralized fibrocartilage, mineralized fibrocartilage, and bone. After repair, the tendon heals to bone with an interposed layer of fibrovascular scar tissue that persists (**Fig. 2**A and B).[7–9] The mechanical properties of this fibrous tissue are weaker than the native insertion site and may render repairs prone to failure.

The Hospital for Special Surgery, Weill Medical College of Cornell University, 535 East 70th Street, New York, NY 10021, USA
* Corresponding author.
E-mail address: rodeos@hss.edu (S.A. Rodeo).

Clin Sports Med 28 (2009) 13–23
doi:10.1016/j.csm.2008.09.002
0278-5919/08/$ – see front matter © 2008 Elsevier Inc. All rights reserved.

sportsmed.theclinics.com

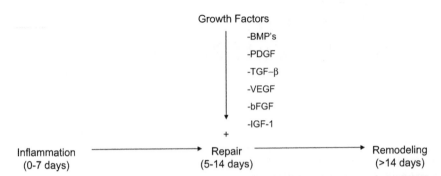

Fig. 1. The stages of rotator cuff healing involve inflammation, repair, and remodeling. Growth factors are expressed during the repair phase, because they promote cell proliferation and matrix production. This timeline must be kept in mind in growth factor therapies, because the addition of growth factors too early or late in the healing process may decrease their effectiveness.

In an effort to limit failures, researchers have focused on ways to minimize the formation of scar tissue at the interface, while at the same time promoting the regeneration of the fibrocartilaginous insertion zones. Initial studies have focused on improving the biomechanical strength of the repair through stronger sutures and by recreating the surface area of the footprint through double-row repairs or their equivalent. Even with these techniques, re-tears or failed healing still occur in up to 12% of patients.[4] Although improved biomechanics may modestly improve healing, it appears that biologic augmentation of the healing process is needed to further reduce failure rates. Biologic therapies that can limit the amount of scar tissue formation at the repair site, and help regenerate a normal fibrocartilaginous transition zone, may theoretically improve the strength of repairs.

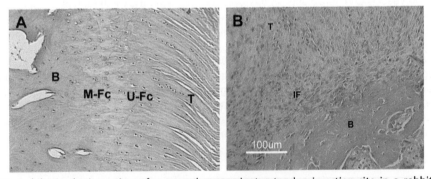

Fig. 2. (*A*) Histologic section of a normal supraspinatus tendon-insertion site in a rabbit, demonstrating the 4 zones of a direct insertion. T, tendon; U-Fc, unmineralized fibrocartilage; M-Fc, mineralized fibrocartilage; B, bone. (*B*) Histologic sections of the tendon-bone attachment site 4 wk after supraspinatus tendon repair in a rat. The resulting attachment site is characterized by a fibrovascular scar tissue interface (IF), without formation of an intermediate zone of fibrocartilage between tendon (T) and bone (B). (*Reprinted from Rodeo SA. Biologic augmentation of rotator cuff tendon repair. J Shoulder Elbow Surg 2007;16(5S):19lS–7S; with permission.*)

Growth factors play an important role in cell chemotaxis, proliferation, matrix synthesis, and cell differentiation. Several growth factors are upregulated during the rotator cuff healing process. Basic fibroblast growth factor (bFGF), bone morphogenetic protein 12 (BMP-12), BMP-13, BMP-14, cartilage oligomeric matrix protein (COMP), connective tissue growth factor (CTGF), platelet-derived growth factor beta (PDGF-B), and transforming growth factor-beta 1 (TGF-β1) have all been shown to be upregulated during the normal healing process of a rat supraspinatus tendon.[10] Because these factors are present during the normal repair process of rotator cuff healing, the theory is that exogenous addition of these factors can further augment the healing process, much as BMP-2 and 7 have done for bone healing.

Several challenges exist in developing an effective biologic therapy to augment rotator cuff healing. First, the most effective growth factor or combination of growth factors must be determined. As research progresses, it is clear that a single factor therapy may not be sufficient. Rather, it is probable that several factors may be necessary, and the various possible combinations are numerous.

The second challenge is determining the optimum time for growth factor delivery. Growth factors are upregulated during the healing process in a temporal fashion, with most growth factors being upregulated 1 week following repair in rat models.[10–12] In the first week after injury/repair, the healing process is in the inflammatory phase. It is possible that this inflammatory response may override any anabolic agent that is added at this time. Therefore, timing of growth factor application is critical. This is supported by a study by Chan and colleagues[13] in which they found that addition of PDGF into a rat patellar tendon defect at 3 days had no effect on the biomechanical strength of the repair, whereas PDGF injection on day 7 improved peak loads-to-failure. Therefore, any growth factor added at the time of surgery needs to be incorporated into a sustained-release drug delivery vehicle that ensures that the factor is present during the regenerative phase of healing.

The final challenge involves developing a delivery vehicle for the growth factor. Many rotator cuff repair surgeries are now performed arthroscopically, so the delivery vehicle must be amenable to placement through cannulas and the growth factor must not be eluted in the fluid-filled arthroscopic environment. These technical considerations make gels, pastes, cements, and glues less desirable than scaffolds or patches.

In this review, the most recent research into the ability of growth factors to augment rotator cuff healing is discussed. Because healing depends on tendon-to-bone healing at the footprint, as well as tendon-to-tendon healing for side-to-side repairs, investigations that examine both processes are discussed. This is followed by a brief review on novel advances for the delivery of growth factors to the repair site. At the conclusion of the review, the reader should have an understanding of the various growth factors that have been highlighted as being potentially clinically useful, an appreciation for the recent research into delivery modalities, and the challenges of growth factor therapy for augmentation of rotator cuff repair.

STUDIES ON THE APPLICATION OF GROWTH FACTORS TO IMPROVE HEALING

In animal models, growth factors are effective in increasing the cellularity and overall tissue volume at the repair site. These findings usually result in increased failure loads on biomechanical testing; however, these failure loads become less significant when they are normalized to the volume or cross-sectional area of the repaired tissue. This implies that growth factors are able to improve the strength of the repair by promoting the formation of more scar tissue (ie, the structural properties are improved but the material properties are not improved). Excessive scar tissue at the healing attachment site may predispose patients to impingement postoperatively. The ultimate outcome of the repair depends on both pullout strength and stiffness. Stiffness and creep may be more important parameters. Ideally, biologic therapies are able to induce tissue formation with material properties close to that of normal tissue.

Osteoinductive Proteins

Secure healing between tendon and bone requires bone ingrowth into the fibrovascular scar tissue and outer tendon. Therefore, factors that induce bone formation may theoretically improve the strength of the repair. Several studies have used this strategy to improve tendon healing in a bone tunnel in animal models, analogous to an anterior cruciate ligament (ACL) repair. However, there are few studies on improving rotator cuff repairs with osteoinductive factors. Rodeo and colleagues[14] studied the effects of an osteoinductive bone protein extract derived from bovine cortical bone (Sulzer Biologics, Wheat Ridge, CO) in a sheep model. This extract contains BMPs 2 through 7, TGF-β1, TGF-β2, TGF-β3, and FGF. The experimental group received 1.0 mg of the bone protein extract on a type-I collagen sponge, which was placed between the infraspinatus and the bone before repair and animals were sacrificed at 6 weeks and 12 weeks. Based on magnetic resonance imaging, repairs that received the bone-protein extract had a greater volume of bone and soft tissue at the repair site at both time points when compared with controls. Histologic examination showed significantly more fibrocartilage between the tendon and the bone in the experimental group. The imaging and histology results correlated with greater failure loads at both 6 and 12 weeks in the treated group. However, when the failure loads were normalized by tissue volume, there were no differences between groups. This suggests that growth factor treatment resulted in the formation of poor-quality scar tissue rather than true tissue regeneration.

Bone Morphogenetic Proteins-12 and -13 (BMP-12 and -13)

BMP-12 (also known as growth and differentiation factor 7) and BMP-13 (growth and differentiation factor 6) are both expressed at the embryonic development sites that form tendons and their insertions.[15] These molecules are distinct from the osteoinductive BMPs (BMP-2,-4,-7) and induce formation of tendon and fibrocartilage. Studies have reported that administration of recombinant human BMP-12 (rhBMP-12) and rhBMP-13 leads to induction of neo-tendon/ligament formation in rats and improved healing of tendon laceration.[15–17] A study conducted in conjunction with Wyeth Research, Inc., investigated the effects of rhBMP-12 (Wyeth Research, Cambridge, MA) on rotator cuff tendon-bone healing in a sheep model.[18] In this study, 4 treatment groups were evaluated: rhBMP-12 in injectable hyaluronan paste, rhBMP-12 in hyaluronan sponge, rhBMP-12 in absorbable type-I collagen sponge, and rhBMP-12 type-I/III collagen sponge. These were compared with a control group that underwent detachment and repair of the infraspinatus. At 8 weeks, specimens treated with rhBMP-12 in collagen sponges were 2.7 times stronger than untreated specimens, whereas those treated with rhBMP-12 in hyaluronan sponges were 2.1 times stronger than controls. Interestingly, specimens treated with rhBMP-12 in hyaluronan paste were similar to untreated controls, again demonstrating the importance of the delivery vehicle in growth factor therapy. Histologic evaluation found reestablishment of collagen fiber continuity between the bone and the fibrovascular interface scar tissue, with increased glycosaminoglycan content in the rhBMP-12-treated specimens. These results suggest that rhBMP-12 may be useful in improving rotator cuff repair healing.

Platelet-Derived Growth Factor

PDGF-BB has been found to act as a mitogen and chemotactic cytokine that can potentially enhance ligament and tendon healing. In a rat model of knee medial ligament (MCL) healing after transection, it was found that treatment with PDGF alone when compared with a combination of growth factors improved the structural properties of the femoral-MCL-tibial complexes.[19] In a rabbit knee medial collateral ligament rupture model, the application of PDGF-BB delivered in fibrin sealant significantly improved the ultimate load, energy absorbed to failure, and ultimate elongation values of the femur–MCL–tibia complex when compared with the control group.[20] In a rat patellar-tendon defect model, there was an increased proliferative response when PDGF-BB was supplemented on day 3 after surgery by way of syringe injection, whereas supplementation on day 7 improved peak load and pyridinoline content after administration of the highest dosage of PDGF.[13] In a rat model of rotator cuff repair, delivery of cells expressing PDGF-BB with a polyglycolic acid (PGA) scaffold showed restoration of normal crimp patterning and collagen bundle alignment compared with suture repair only.[21] A study conducted in the authors' laboratory evaluated the ability of PDGF-BB on a collagen scaffold to improve rotator cuff healing in a rat. Increased cellular proliferation and angiogenesis were found in a dose-dependant fashion at 5 days; however, this did not correlate with improved healing at 28 days based on histology or biomechanical testing.[22] These studies demonstrate that improved healing with PDGF is dependent on the dosage, timing, and delivery vehicle used.

There are currently several commercially available systems to create a "platelet-rich plasma" or "platelet gel" from autologous blood. These systems involve spinning autologous blood in a centrifuge to form a dense, suturable fibrin matrix that can be easily placed directly at the tendon repair site. One technical problem with these systems is that many use human or bovine thrombin to form the platelet-rich plasma. Excess thrombin causes premature platelet activation and degranulation, causing immediate release of the platelet-derived cytokines. Newer systems have omitted the use of thrombin to prevent this phenomenon during processing. Currently, there are no clinical studies on the efficacy of this treatment though theoretically it holds promise.

Transforming Growth Factor-β

During wound healing, TGF-β is released from degranulating platelets and secreted by all the major cell types participating in the healing process, including lymphocytes, macrophages, endothelial cells, smooth muscle cells, epithelial cells, and fibroblasts.[23] Scar tissue formation has been closely associated with the presence of the 3 TGF-β isoforms (TBF-β1, 2, and 3). Although adult wounds heal with an abundance of scar tissue, which is correlated with increased expression of TGF- β1, fetal wounds heal without scar and without expression of TBF-β1. Therefore, inhibition of TGF-β1 or exogenous application of TGF-β3 may reduce scar tissue formation in the interface. TBF-β3 is expressed during fetal tendon development. In a study on a rat rotator cuff repair model, Kim and colleagues[24] found that exogenous application of TGF-β3 resulted in improved mechanical properties when compared to specimens treated with TGF-β1. Conversely, application of TGF-β1 coupled with suppression of TGF-β2 and -3 led to mechanically inferior tissue despite increased cross-sectional area. This suggests that although TGF-β1 results in the exuberant production of scar tissue at the repair site, this tissue is mechanically weaker than normal tissue. The ultimate goal in developing strategies to improve rotator cuff healing is to limit the amount of scar formation, while maximizing the strength of the repair.

Vascular Endothelial Growth Factor

It is well established that the rotator cuff tendon is hypovascular in the area adjacent to the distal insertion site.[1] Therefore, it seems reasonable that increased vascularity could improve rotator cuff healing. VEGF is known to have a potent angiogenic effect and is expressed in high concentration in healing flexor tendons 7 to 10 days following repair, with a return to normal by 14 days.[10] No studies have directly evaluated the role of these molecules in rotator cuff repair. However, Zhang and colleagues[25] injected VEGF into repaired Achilles tendons in a rat model and found improved tensile strength early in the course of healing. In contrast, a recent study on the ability of VEGF on graft healing in a sheep ACL reconstruction model showed no benefit in VEGF therapy over controls.[26] In this study, the grafts were soaked in VEGF in the experimental group, whereas the control group grafts were soaked in phosphate buffered saline. Although there was increased vascularity in the VEGF-treated group, the stiffness of the femur–graft–tibia complex in the VEGF-treated group was significantly lower than in controls. Although only a single concentration of VEGF solution was used, and the animals were evaluated at only 1 time point (12 weeks), these preliminary data suggest that excessive vascularity may have detrimental effects on the healing ACL graft. It is unclear if these findings can be extrapolated to rotator cuff healing.

Basic Fibroblast Growth Factor

bFGF causes fibroblasts to produce collagenase and stimulates proliferation of capillary endothelial cells, both of which are necessary for angiogenesis. It also helps to initiate the formation of granulation tissue. In vitro work has shown bFGF results in cell proliferation and collagen production in cultured flexor-tendon tenocytes.[27,28]

Recent in vivo work also appears encouraging, though there are no studies to date that have evaluated bFGF in a rotator cuff repair model. Chan and colleagues[29] injected bFGF in various doses into rat patella tendons 3 days after a window defect was created. At 7 days, there was a dose-dependent increase in the number of proliferating cells and the level of expression of type-III collagen. However, these results were not seen at 14 days, nor were there any differences in the ultimate stress and the pyridinoline content of the healing tendons. Tang and colleagues[30] used a digital flexor-tendon repair model in chickens to evaluate the efficacy of injecting bFGF in an adeno-associated viral vector into the lacerated tendon ends before repair. They found that tendons treated with this vector had increased ultimate loads-to-failure when compared with those treated with a sham vector, or no vector at all, at 2, 4, and 8 weeks. Exogenous bFGF loaded onto a monofilament nylon suture has also been shown to result in more cellularity and increased failure loads at 3 weeks in another flexor-tendon repair model.[31]

Insulin-Like Growth Factor-1

IGF-1 has been shown to have anabolic effects on healing tendons by stimulating protein synthesis, increasing cell proliferation, collagen synthesis, and decreasing swelling. In vitro studies have shown that the addition of IGF-1 to tenocytes in culture induces matrix synthesis, but did not affect matrix turnover.[28] Kurtz and colleagues[32] applied exogenous IGF-1 to repaired rat Achilles tendons and found that it stimulated the synthesis of DNA, collagen, and proteoglycans and that this resulted in reduced time to functional recovery. Dines et al. studied the ability of rat tendon fibroblasts transduced with a retroviral vector containing IGF-1.[33] These cells were then seeded onto a bioabsorbable polymer scaffold that was made of nonwoven, PGA. The scaffold was then tested in a rat rotator cuff model. At 6 weeks, specimens treated with the IGF-1 seeded scaffold exhibited better histology scores and a higher ultimate load-to-failure than those with the scaffold alone. This study introduced a novel manner by which to deliver growth factors to the healing repair site, and its results are encouraging and warrant further investigation in larger animal models.

DEVELOPMENTAL BIOLOGY AS A PARADIGM FOR TENDON REGENERATION

Work in developmental biology laboratories have identified several molecules that are thought to play a role in tendon and tendon-bone development during embryogenesis. The theory is that an understanding of the mechanisms by which tendons and tendon-bone interfaces are formed in the fetus will one day lead to therapies that can induce regeneration of normal tissue as opposed to the fibrosis seen in adults. Scleraxis is a transcription factor that is upregulated in tissues that develop into tendons, leading researchers to postulate that it plays a role in driving tenocyte differentiation.[34] Shukanami and colleagues[35] linked scleraxis expression with another tenocyte marker, a transmembrane glycoprotein named tenomodulin. The role these proteins play in the formation of tendons is still unclear, but they have been shown to result in tenocyte proliferation. There have been no in vivo studies investigating their ability to improve rotator cuff healing.

Initial formation of tendons occurs independently with respect to muscle, but later development depends on signals from the muscle to drive tendon development and maturation. FGF-4 is secreted from the muscle of developing chick embryos. Its presence results in upregulation of scleraxis and another tendon marker, tenascin.[36] This implies that FGF-4 may be responsible for proliferation of tenocytes and maturation of tendons during development. Another protein necessary for tendon development is myostatin (GDF-8). Mendias and colleagues[37] showed that the tendons of myostatin knockout mice were smaller, more brittle, had less cellularity, and had a decrease in the expression of type-I collagen. Conversely, treatment of tendon fibroblasts with myostatin activated tenocyte proliferation pathways and increased the production of type-I collagen. Although the field of tendon development and its translational application to the augmentation of rotator cuff repairs is in its infancy, the possible therapies this research can lead to is exciting.

GROWTH FACTOR DELIVERY METHODS

Perhaps the most challenging aspect of growth factor therapy for the augmentation of rotator cuff repairs is determining a way to deliver the factor to the healing site. As discussed, once the proper combination of growth factors has been determined, as well as their optimal time for delivery, they then need to be delivered to the tendon-bone healing site in a fluid-filled arthroscopic environment without interfering with healing. Gene therapy approaches and tissue regenerative scaffolds are currently being investigated.

Gene Therapy

Gene therapy was first developed to treat inherited genetic defects by replacing a defective copy of the gene with a normal one. In orthopedics, however, attention has been turned to this technique as a biologic sustained release, local growth factor delivery vehicle. There are 2 main strategies for growth factor delivery with gene therapy, "ex vivo" and "in vivo" (**Fig. 3**).[38] The ex vivo technique involves transferring the gene that codes for the growth factor of interest into carrier cells in vitro. These cells then overexpress the growth factor for which the gene codes for and releases it into the

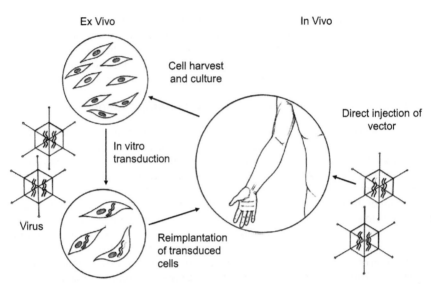

Fig. 3. The 2 basic gene therapy strategies: in vivo and ex vivo. The in vivo strategy involves administering the vector containing the gene of interest directly to the patient. The ex vivo method involves harvesting cells, transducing them with the vector containing the gene in vitro, then re-administering the cells into the repair site. (*Reprinted from* Musgrave DS, Fu FH, Huard J. Gene therapy and tissue engineering in orthopaedic surgery. J Am Acad Orthop Surg 2002;10:6–15; with permission.)

local environment. The transduced stem cells are then added to the repair site where they release the growth factor for an extended period of time. The second, less common, method involves delivering the gene of interest directly into the local cells of the healing tissue. This involves exposing the host tissue to the vector containing the gene of interest. This technique is less attractive because the vector is usually a virus, and there is a risk of contaminating the surrounding tissue and the surgeon.

Tissue Engineering Scaffolds and Coated Sutures

Scaffolds are 3-dimensional structures that promote regeneration of the surrounding tissue. The scaffold by itself may guide new tissue formation by its 3-dimensional architecture. It may also be seeded with either cells, growth factors, or both. Scaffolds can be made of naturally derived polymers, such as collagen and hyaluronic acid, synthetic polymers, such as polyL-lactic acid (PLLA), PGA, polyDL-lactic-co-glycolic acid (PLGA), polyvinyl alcohol (PVA), or injectable polymers that cross-link in situ, such as alginate and polyethylene oxide (PEO). In the simplest design, the various scaffolds can be soaked in a solution containing the growth factor such that the factor wicks onto it. This scaffold can then be added to the repair site where the growth factor is eluted into the local environment. This technique has been outlined by Dines and colleagues,[39] in which a Vicryl (polyglactin 910, Ethicon, Somerville, NJ) was coated with rhGDF-5. They showed that a consistent amount of growth factor is released from the sutures after passage through soft tissue.

More complex strategies have also been outlined in which hydrogels are embedded with microspheres that contain growth factors. The microspheres then are able to release the factor at a controlled rate. This technique offers the option to load the scaffold with more than 1 growth factor. Furthermore, the microspheres can be engineered to release different growth factors at different rates, so that the factors can be released in a temporal fashion. Although research in this field has progressed substantially, these technologies are still far from being clinically useful.

SUMMARY

The 4 fibrocartilaginous transition zones of the rotator cuff insertion site are not recreated following surgical repair. Instead, a layer of scar tissue is formed between the tendon and the bone, which renders repairs prone to failure. Growth factors are a group of cytokines that induce mitosis, extracellular matrix production, neovascularization, cell maturation, and differentiation. Research has focused on their ability to augment rotator cuff repairs. Studies have shown that several factors are capable of increasing the strength of repairs in animal models. However, this appears to be accomplished through the production of more scar tissue, as opposed to regeneration of native tissue. It is becoming clear that multiple factors may be needed to regenerate the native tendon-bone insertion site. The optimal timing and vehicle for growth factor deliver have remained elusive. Gene therapy and tissue scaffolds provide promising options for the future, but the engineering still needs to be optimized for clinical use. Growth factor therapy for rotator cuff repairs remains a promising therapeutic for the future; however, much work needs to be done to optimize its effectiveness.

REFERENCES

1. Fealy S, Adler RS, Drakos MC, et al. Patterns of vascular and anatomical response after rotator cuff repair. Am J Sports Med 2006;34(1):120–7.
2. Galatz LM, Ball CM, Teefey SA, et al. The outcome and repair integrity of completely arthroscopically repaired large and massive rotator cuff tears. J Bone Joint Surg Am 2004;86A(2):219–24.
3. Harryman DT 2nd, Mack LA, Wang KY, et al. Repairs of the rotator cuff. Correlation of functional results with integrity of the cuff. J Bone Joint Surg Am 1991; 73(7):982–9.
4. Lafosse L, Brozska R, Toussaint B, et al. The outcome and structural integrity of arthroscopic rotator cuff repair with use of the double-row suture anchor technique. J Bone Joint Surg Am 2007;89(7):1533–41.
5. Gerber C, Fuchs B, Hodler J. The results of repair of massive tears of the rotator cuff. J Bone Joint Surg Am 2000;82(4):505–15.
6. Boileau P, Brassart N, Watkinson DJ, et al. Arthroscopic repair of full-thickness tears of the supraspinatus: does the tendon really heal? J Bone Joint Surg Am 2005;87(6):1229–40.
7. Carpenter JE, Thomopoulos S, Flanagan CL, et al. Rotator cuff defect healing: a biomechanical and histologic analysis in an animal model. J Shoulder Elbow Surg 1998;7(6):599–605.
8. Cohen DB, Kawamura S, Ehteshami JR, et al. Indomethacin and celecoxib impair rotator cuff tendon-to-bone healing. Am J Sports Med 2006;34(3):362–9.
9. Galatz LM, Sandell LJ, Rothermich SY, et al. Characteristics of the rat supraspinatus tendon during tendon-to-bone healing after acute injury. J Orthop Res 2006;24(3):541–50.
10. Wurgler-Hauri CC, Dourte LM, Baradet TC, et al. Temporal expression of 8 growth factors in tendon-to-bone healing in a rat supraspinatus model. J Shoulder Elbow Surg 2007;16(Suppl 5):S198–203.
11. Kobayashi M, Itoi E, Minagawa H, et al. Expression of growth factors in the early phase of supraspinatus tendon healing in rabbits. J Shoulder Elbow Surg 2006; 15(3):371–7.

12. Dahlgren LA, Mohammed HO, Nixon AJ. Temporal expression of growth factors and matrix molecules in healing tendon lesions. J Orthop Res 2005;23(1): 84–92.
13. Chan BP, Fu SC, Qin L, et al. Supplementation-time dependence of growth factors in promoting tendon healing. Clin Orthop Relat Res 2006;448:240–7.
14. Rodeo SA, Potter HG, Kawamura S, et al. Biologic augmentation of rotator cuff tendon-healing with use of a mixture of osteoinductive growth factors. J Bone Joint Surg Am 2007;89(11):2485–97.
15. Wolfman NM, Hattersley G, Cox K, et al. Ectopic induction of tendon and ligament in rats by growth and differentiation factors 5, 6, and 7, members of the TGF-beta gene family. J Clin Invest 1997;100(2):321–30.
16. Lou J, Tu Y, Burns M, et al. BMP-12 gene transfer augmentation of lacerated tendon repair. J Orthop Res 2001;19(6):1199–202.
17. Aspenberg P, Forslund C. Enhanced tendon healing with GDF 5 and 6. Acta Orthop Scand 1999;70(1):51–4.
18. Seeherman HJ, Archambault JM, Rodeo SA, et al. rhBMP-12 accelerates healing of rotator cuff repairs in a sheep model. J Bone Joint Surg Am 2008;90:2206–19.
19. Letson AK, Dahners LE. The effect of combinations of growth factors on ligament healing. Clin Orthop Relat Res 1994;308:207–12.
20. Hildebrand KA, Woo SL, Smith DW, et al. The effects of platelet-derived growth factor-BB on healing of the rabbit medial collateral ligament. An in vivo study. Am J Sports Med 1998;26(4):549–54.
21. Uggen JC, Dines J, Uggen CW, et al. Tendon gene therapy modulates the local repair environment in the shoulder. J Am Osteopath Assoc 2005; 105(1):20–1.
22. Kovacevic D, Gulotta L, Nickols J, et al. PDGF induces cell proliferation and angiogenesis in a rat rotator cuff repair model of tendon-bone healing. Presented at the Annual Meeting of the American Orthopaedic Society for Sports Medicine, Orlando (FL), July 10–13, 2008.
23. Molloy T, Wang Y, Murrell G. The roles of growth factors in tendon and ligament healing. Sports Med 2003;33(5):381–94.
24. Kim HM, Galatz L, Das R, et al. The role of TGF-Beta during tendon to bone healing. Trans of the Orthopaedic Research Society 2006;31:1060.
25. Zhang F, Liu H, Stile F, et al. Effect of vascular endothelial growth factor on rat achilles tendon healing. Plast Reconstr Surg 2003;112(6):1613–9.
26. Yoshikawa T, Tohyama H, Katsura T, et al. Effects of local administration of vascular endothelial growth factor on mechanical characteristics of the semitendinosus tendon graft after anterior cruciate ligament reconstruction in sheep. Am J Sports Med 2006;34(12):1918–25.
27. Takahasih S, Nakajima M, Kobayashi M, et al. Effect of recombinant basic fibroblast growth factor (bFGF) on fibroblast-like cells from human rotator cuff tendon. Tohoku J Exp Med 2002;198(4):207–14.
28. Thomopoulos S, Harwood FL, Silva MJ, et al. Effect of several growth factors on canine flexor tendon fibroblast proliferation and collagen synthesis in vitro. J Hand Surg [Am] 2005;30(3):441–7.
29. Chan BP, Fu S, Qin L, et al. Effects of basic fibroblast growth factor (bFGF) on early stages of tendon healing: a rat patellar tendon model. Acta Orthop Scand 2000;71(5):513–8.
30. Tang JB, Cao Y, Zhu B, et al. Adeno-associated virus-2-mediated bFGF gene transfer to digital flexor tendons significantly increases healing strength. An in vivo study. J Bone Joint Surg Am 2008;90(5):1078–89.

31. Hamada Y, Katoh S, Hibino N, et al. Effects of monofilament nylon coated with basic fibroblast growth factor on endogenous intrasynovial flexor tendon healing. J Hand Surg [Am] 2006;31(4):530–40.
32. Kurtz CA, Loebig TG, Anderson DD, et al. Insulin-like growth factor I accelerates functional recovery from achilles tendon injury in a rat model. Am J Sports Med 1999;27(3):363–9.
33. Dines JS, Grande DA, Dines DM. Tissue engineering and rotator cuff tendon healing. J Shoulder Elbow Surg 2007;16(5 Suppl):S204–7.
34. Pryce BA, Brent AE, Murchison ND, et al. Generation of transgenic tendon reporters, ScxGFP and ScxAP, using regulatory elements of the scleraxis gene. Dev Dyn 2007;236(6):1677–82.
35. Shukunami C, Takimoto A, Oro M, et al. Scleraxis positively regulates the expression of tenomodulin, a differentiation marker of tenocytes. Dev Biol 2006;298(1):234–47.
36. Edom-Vovard F, Schuler B, Bonnin MA, et al. Fgf4 positively regulates scleraxis and tenascin expression in chick limb tendons. Dev Biol 2002;247(2):351–66.
37. Mendias CL, Bakhurin KI, Faulkner JA. Tendons of myostatin-deficient mice are small, brittle, and hypocellular. Proc Natl Acad Sci U S A 2008;105(1):388–93.
38. Musgrave DS, Fu FH, Huard J. Gene therapy and tissue engineering in orthopaedic surgery. J Am Acad Orthop Surg 2002;10(1):6–15.
39. Dines JS, Weber L, Razzano P, et al. The effect of growth differentiation factor-5-coated sutures on tendon repair in a rat model. J Shoulder Elbow Surg 2007;16(Suppl 5):S215–21.

Emerging Options for Treatment of Articular Cartilage Injury in the Athlete

Kai Mithoefer, MD[a],*, Timothy R. McAdams, MD[b], Jason M. Scopp, MD[c], Bert R. Mandelbaum, MD[d]

KEYWORDS

- Cartilage - Repair - Novel - Sports athlete
- Reconstruction - Return to sport

INCIDENCE OF ATHLETIC CARTILAGE INJURY

Injuries of the articular cartilage surfaces of the knee are frequently observed in athletes. Although no study has systematically investigated the incidence of sports-related articular cartilage injury, an increasing number of chondral injuries in high-impact sports has been observed, particularly at the competitive collegiate, professional, and world-class level.[1] Besides this rising incidence in high-level competitive sports, increasing recreational participation in pivoting sports such as football, basketball, and soccer has been associated with a rising number of sports-related articular cartilage injuries.[2–4] Injuries of the articular cartilage surface of the knee in the athlete frequently result in association with other acute injuries, such as ligament or meniscal injuries, traumatic patellar dislocations, and osteochondral injuries.[4–6] Articular cartilage defects of the femoral condyles have been observed in up to 50% of athletes undergoing anterior cruciate ligament reconstruction, with increased propensity in female athletes.[6,7] Besides acute injury, articular cartilage defects can develop in the high-impact athletic population from chronic pathologic joint-loading patterns, such as joint instability or malalignment.[4–6] Irrespective of their origin, articular cartilage injuries in athletes will frequently limit the ability of the affected athletes to continue participation in their sport and predispose them to progressive joint degeneration.[8,9]

[a] Harvard Vanguard Orthopedics and Sports Medicine, Harvard Medical School, Boston, MA, USA
[b] Stanford University, Department of Orthopaedic Surgery, Palo Alto, CA, USA
[c] Peninsula Orthopedic Associates, 1675 Woodbrooke Drive, Salisbury, MD 21804, USA
[d] Santa Monica Orthopedic and Sports Medicine Foundation, Los Angeles, CA, USA
* Corresponding author.
E-mail address: kmithoefer@partners.org (K. Mithoefer).

Clin Sports Med 28 (2009) 25–40
doi:10.1016/j.csm.2008.09.001
0278-5919/08/$ – see front matter

NATURAL HISTORY OF ATHLETIC CARTILAGE INJURY

The limited spontaneous repair following acute or chronic articular cartilage injury is well documented.[10–12] The lack of vascularization of articular cartilage prevents the physiologic inflammatory response to tissue injury and resultant repair. This failure of recruitment of extrinsic undifferentiated repair cells combined with the intrinsic inability for replication and repair by the mature chondrocytes results in a repaired cartilage that is both qualitatively and quantitatively insufficient. Furthermore, repetitive loading of the injured articular cartilage, such as in impact and pivoting sports, results in further cellular degeneration with accumulation of degradative enzymes and cytokines, disruption of collagen ultrastructure, increased hydration, and fissuring of the articular surface. These biochemical and metabolic changes are similar to the changes seen in early osteoarthritis.[13]

Although experimental studies have provided much insight into the mechanisms involved in the progression of cartilage injury to osteoarthritis, there is still limited prospective clinical information about the natural history of articular cartilage lesions, particularly in athletes. In a long-term study of 28 Swedish athletes with isolated severe chondral damage in the weight-bearing condyles, 75% of athletes returned to their sport initially, but a significant decline in athletic activity was observed 14 years after the initial injury, with radiographic evidence of osteoarthritis in 57% of these athletes.[14] Similar poor results were reported in a prospective study of untreated osteochondral defects in 38% of athletically active patients, with moderate to severe radiographic evidence of osteoarthritis in 45% at 34 years after diagnosis.[15] One recent report in athletes with anterior cruciate ligament (ACL) injuries demonstrated that hyaline cartilage defects in these patients resulted in significant pain and swelling and were associated with marked lifestyle changes and limitation of athletic activity.[16] Similarly, other studies have shown that untreated articular cartilage defects in patients with ACL deficiency resulted in significantly worse outcome scores up to 19 years after the original injury.[17] These results are supported by the 4- to 5-fold increased risk of knee osteoarthritis in high-demand, pivoting athletes established by the National Institute of Health (NIH) and in several other independent studies.[8,9,18–21]

ATHLETIC ACTIVITY AND CHONDROPENIA

Intact articular cartilage possesses optimal load-bearing characteristics and adjusts to the level of activity. Increasing weight-bearing activity in athletes and adolescents has been shown to increase the volume and thickness of articular cartilage.[22] In the healthy athlete, a positive linear dose–response relationship exists for repetitive loading activities and articular cartilage function. However, recent studies indicate that this dose–response curve reaches a threshold and that activity beyond this threshold can result in maladaptation and injury of articular cartilage.[23] High-impact joint loading above this threshold has been shown to decrease cartilage protoglycan content, increase levels of degradative enzymes, and cause chondrocyte apoptosis.[12,13,24] If the integrity of the functional weight bearing unit is lost, either through acute injury or chronic microtrauma in the high-impact athlete, a chondropenic response is initiated, which can include loss of articular cartilage volume and stiffness, elevation of contact pressures, and development or progression of articular cartilage defects. Concomitant pathologic factors, such as ligamentous instability, malalignment, meniscal injury, or deficiency, can further support progression of the chondropenic cascade. Without intervention, chondropenia contributes to the deterioration of articular cartilage function in high-impact athletes and may ultimately progress to osteoarthritis.

TREATMENT OPTIONS FOR ATHLETIC CARTILAGE INJURY

The high demands on the joint surfaces in athletes and high risk for joint degeneration make treatment of articular cartilage injuries and restoration of the injured joint surfaces critically important to facilitate continued athletic participation and to maintain a physically active lifestyle. Maintaining an active lifestyle is important not only from an orthopedic standpoint but has also several significant medical benefits, such as reducing the risk for serious medical conditions such as heart disease, hypertension, and diabetes. Because injuries to articular cartilage of the knee have been shown to present one of the most common causes of permanent disability in athletes, management of articular cartilage in this high-demand population has important long-term implications.[18–21] Due to the documented detrimental effect of high-impact articular loading, articular cartilage repair in the athletic population requires cartilage surface restoration, which can withstand the significant mechanical joint stresses generated during high-impact, pivoting sports.[11,12] Besides reducing pain, increasing mobility, and improving knee function, the ability to return the athlete to sport and to enable the athlete to continue to perform at the pre-injury athletic level presents one of the most important parameters for a successful outcome from articular cartilage repair in this challenging population.

Treatment of articular cartilage injuries in the athletic population has traditionally presented a significant therapeutic challenge.[11,25] However, the development of new surgical techniques has created considerable clinical and scientific enthusiasm for articular cartilage repair.[25–29] Based on the source of the cartilage repair tissue, these new surgical techniques can generally be categorized into 3 groups: marrow stimulation-based techniques, osteochondral transplantation techniques, and cell-based repair techniques. Prospective clinical results of these techniques are still limited.[30,31] Each of the new cartilage repair techniques is associated with unique advantages and limitations. New treatment options are being developed that integrate modern tissue engineering and genetic augmentation techniques to further improve quantity and quality of the repair cartilage generated by the currently existing cartilage restoration methods.

Marrow Stimulation Techniques

Microfracture
Due to its limited invasiveness, low associated morbidity, and relatively short postoperative rehabilitation, microfracture has become a popular treatment option for articular cartilage lesions in the athlete's knee. By micropenetration of the subchondral plate, this technique results in filling the cartilage defect by a blood clot that contains pluripotent marrow-derived mesenchymal stem cells (MSCs), which subsequently produce a mixed fibrocartilage repair tissue that contains varying amounts of type II collagen.[32,33] Improved knee function has been reported in 58% to 95% athletes after microfracture with significantly increased activity scores.[34–37] Return to competition was demonstrated in 44% to 77% of athletes after microfracture, with 57% of them at the preoperative level.[34–37]

Several factors have been shown to affect the results from microfracture in athletes. The time between injury and microfracture has significant influence on outcome with players, emphasizing the critical role of early surgical treatment of articular cartilage lesions for successful return to demanding sports.[36,37] Microfracture is most effective as a first-line procedure in athletes younger than 40 years and lesion size ≤ 200 mm^2.[37,38] Following initial functional improvement, deterioration of knee function has been described in 47% to 80% of athletes after 24 months.[34,36–38] Although the exact reason for this functional decline is not known, some studies suggest that repair cartilage volume plays a critical role for durability, because deterioration of knee function occurs primarily with poor repair cartilage fill.[38,39] Postoperative magnetic resonance imaging (MRI) demonstrates depressed repair cartilage morphology and incomplete peripheral integration in 53% to 96% and subchondral bony overgrowth in 25% to 40%.[38,39] Lack of peripheral integration and relative thinning of the repair cartilage increases mechanical stresses on the repair cartilage and promotes repair cartilage degeneration and may contribute to the observed functional deterioration in the demanding athletic population.

Enhanced microfracture techniques

Despite its current limitations, recent data has shown that the microfracture technique provides multipotent stem cell-like mesenchymal progenitor cells with a high chondrogenic differentiation potential.[40] This has prompted investigation of new technologies that can help to enhance the results from the first-generation microfracture technique. In experimental studies, the addition of growth factors such as transforming growth factor-β3 (TGF-β3) and bone morphogenetic protein 7 (BMP-7) was able to induce chondrogenic marker gene expression for type II and IX collagen, cartilage oligometric matrix protein (COMP), and aggrecan with both qualitative and quantitative improvement of the repair cartilage after microfracture.[40,41] Besides directly stimulating chondrogenic differentiation, a different approach involves enhancement of the microfracture repair by modulation of the potential negative effect of cytokines on the repair tissue. Recent long-term experimental data have shown promise by demonstrating increased proteoglycan and type II collagen content in the microfracture repair tissue after stimulating local production of interleukin-1 receptor antagonist protein (IL-1 ra) by in vivo gene therapy.[42] However, although these approaches are scientifically plausible and the results are promising, their transition to clinical application is still pending. In contrast, clinical evaluation has started for other microfracture-based cartilage repair techniques that use scaffold-guided in situ chondroinduction.[43,44] These technologies use three-dimensional (3-D) scaffolds to enhance the initial stability and peripheral adhesion of the microfracture clot, thereby reducing the risk for early clot displacement. In situ solidification of the microfracture clot with chitosan-glycerol phosphate (BST-CarGel, Bisosyntec Inc, Laval, Quebec, Canada), a thrombogenic and adhesive polysaccharide polymer, has been shown to improve cartilage repair volume and biochemical composition after experimental microfracture.[43,45] Preliminary clinical data from 33 patients have demonstrated the safety of this technique with improvement of WOMAC scores after 12 to 24 months.[46] Other authors have developed a novel method that uses a combination of microfracture with a combination of a multifunctional chondroitin sulfate for peripheral adhesion and injectable biodegradable hydrogel scaffold to enhance microfracture repair (**Fig. 1**) (Cartilix Inc, San Carlos, CA). Photopolymerization of the hydrogel allows for rapid stabilization of the combined cellular implant (**Fig. 1**).[44] In clinical trials, this technique has shown improved repair cartilage volume on MRI at 6 months after implantation compared with microfracture alone (**Fig. 2**). Prospective, randomized long-term comparisons are needed to further evaluate the promising new technologies specifically in the demanding athletic population.

Osteochondral Transfer Techniques

Osteochondral autograft transplantation

The use of osteochondral autografts for repair of focal chondral and osteochondral lesions has been popularized by Hangody.[47] This technique provides a hyaline cartilage

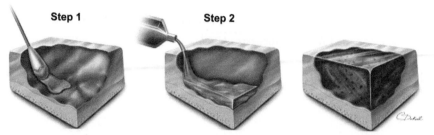

Fig. 1. The principle of the enhanced microfracture technique. Following microfracture of the defect, a chondroitin-sulfate adhesive is applied to the surface of the cartilage defect (Step 1). A pregel macromer solution is added to the defects treated with the adhesive (Step 2). Photopolymerization is then performed resulting in a solid hydrogel that is covalently bound to the cartilage surface through the chondroitin-sulfate bridge. Mesenchymal stem cells from the marrow stimulation can be easily incorporated into the hydrogel layer. (*From* Wang DA, Varghese S, Sharma B, et al. Multifunctional chondroitin sulphate for cartilage tissue-biomaterial integration. Nat Mater 2007;6(5):385–92; with permission.)

repair by harvesting cylindric osteochondral grafts from areas of limited weight bearing and transferring into small to midsize (1–4 cm²) defects of the weight bearing cartilage using a press-fit technique. Two prospective studies have evaluated this technique in athletes with an average time period of 26 to 36 months.[48,49] Up to 95% of patients showed good or excellent results with significantly improved knee function scores. Macroscopic International Cartilage Repair Society (ICRS) scores and MRI demonstrated 84% and 94% good to excellent rating, respectively. Return to athletic activity was reported in 61% to 93% and as early as 6 to 9 months postoperatively. Longer preoperative symptoms and age >30 years were associated with decreased return to sport. Preoperative radiographic or clinical evidence of joint degeneration predicted a return to sport at a lower level or even retirement from competitive sports after osteochondral autograft transfer. Despite the encouraging results, several limitations remain. Restoration of concave or convex articular cartilage surfaces can be technically demanding, and short-term fixation strength and load-bearing capacity may deteriorate early.[50] Incongruity and graft height mismatch can result in significant elevation of contact pressures.[51] Peripheral chondrocyte death from mechanical trauma at the graft and recipient edges can lead to lack of peripheral integration with persistent gap formation.[52,53] Acute donor site morbidity has been described; however, long-term morbidity appears to be low.[48,49,54]

Osteochondral allograft transplantation
Osteochondral allografts have been successfully used for the treatment of large and deep chondral and osteochondral lesions from acute trauma, osteochondritis dissecans, avascular necrosis, and joint degeneration. This technique also provides a hyaline cartilage repair. Because chondrocyte viability, matrix composition, and mechanical properties of hypothermically stored cartilage grafts have been shown to deteriorate rapidly, implantation should be performed as a fresh graft within 28 days of graft harvest.[55] Several studies have shown that the transplanted bone is readily incorporated by the host with good articular cartilage function. However, recent survival analysis revealed deterioration over time, with 95% survival at 5 years, 80% at 10 years, and 65% at 15 years.[56] Better outcomes are seen with unipolar lesions, without malalignment, rigid fixation, and age <60 years.[57] Better outcomes

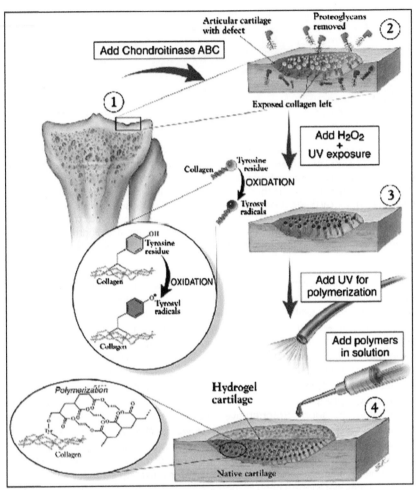

Fig. 2. Graphic demonstrating the sequential process of hydrogel-based enhanced microfracture.

are also seen in young, active adults; however, no study has yet specifically investigated the use of this technique in the athletic population.

Osteochondral graft substitute

To avoid the limitations, morbidity, and potential complications associated with osteochondral auto- or allografts, bioresorbable scaffolds have been developed recently as substitute grafts for treatment of focal chondral and osteochondral defects. These implants are composites of polylactide-glycolide copolymers, calcium sulfate, polyglycolic acid fibers, and surfactant (TruFit, Smith&Nephew Endoscopy, San Antonio, TX). The bilayered cylindric implant is equipped with a bone and cartilage phase, each designed to physically and mechanically match the layers of the adjacent cartilage and subchondral bone. The different biochemical composition and porous nature of each layer facilitate ingrowth of osseous and cartilaginous cells into the bioresorbable implant, which creates a layered neomatrix. Preclinical studies have demonstrated the safety of the implant and the complete resorption of the scaffold with restoration of hyaline-like articular cartilage surfaces and subchondral bone in a high percentage of cases at 12 months. Although no systematic controlled studies are available on this technique, isolated reports have shown favorable results in the treatment after implantation of these osteochondral graft substitutes and even return to high-impact sports.[58,59] However, MRI information at 12 months still demonstrated heterogeneous repair cartilage tissue. and information on long-term durability is not available under the high athletic demands.[59] Besides their use as graft substitutes, these bioresorbable implants can be successfully used for backfill of donor sites in osteochondral autograft transfers.

Cell-Based Cartilage Repair Techniques

Autologous chondocyte transplantation

Successful repair of articular cartilage lesions of the human knee by autologous chondrocyte transplantation was first reported in 1994 by Brittberg who presented the first commercially available cell-based technology (Carticel, Genzyme, Cambridge, MA).[26] Autologous chondrocytes are harvested from a less weight-bearing area of the joint, extracted from the harvested cartilage, and multiplied in vitro before elective reimplantation is performed. Postoperatively, protected weight bearing is maintained for 6 to 8 weeks and return to pivoting sports is usually allowed by 12 months. Autologous chondrocyte transplantation has been successfully used for hyaline-like restoration of full-thickness articular cartilage lesions in the knee by several investigators, with long-term durability of functional improvement of up to 11 years.[60–64] Two recent prospective multi-center studies have evaluated this cartilage repair technique in the athletic population.[63,64] Good to excellent results were demonstrated in 72% to 96%, with improvement of activity scores in 82% to 100%. The best results were obtained with single cartilage lesions of the medial femoral condyle. Thirty-three to ninety-six percent returned to high impact-athletics, 60% to 80% remained at the same skill level. Return to sport was best in competitive athletes (83%) and adolescent athletes (96%) and 87% of returning athletes maintained their ability to perform 52 months after surgery. Athletes with single lesions, age <25 years, and short preoperative intervals had the best rate of return to sport. Participation in sports improved the long-term functional results after autologous chondrocyte transplantation.[65] Limitations of this technique include its invasiveness, long postoperative rehabilitation, and periosteal hypertrophy, which may lead to acute graft delamination.[26,60–64] This cartilage repair technique provides significant functional improvement, with high return rates to demanding sports and excellent durability even under high athletic demands both in the primary and revision setting.

Characterized chondrocyte implantation

In vitro culture and expansion of human chondrocytes for autologous chondrocyte transplantation have been shown to result in a dedifferentiation of the cultured cells, with a shift from a predominantly type II collagen-containing hyaline matrix to a fibrocartilage-like type I collagen-rich repair cartilage.[66] To address this aspect, characterized chondrocyte implantation (CCI) has been developed to improve hyaline articular cartilage regeneration through the identification and selective expansion of specific chondrocyte subpopulations capable of producing more hyaline-like repair cartilage tissue (ChondroCelect, Tigenix, Leuven, Belgium). This subgroup of chondrocytes is characterized by expression of a gene marker profile and phenotypic cell characteristics that have been associated with formation of hyaline cartilage in vivo.[67] Prospective randomized, controlled clinical comparison of CCI with microfracture has shown superior structural repair and histomorphometry with CCI at 12 months.[66] Mid- and long-term results are pending and direct comparison with uncharacterized autologous chondrocyte transplantation is not available.

Scaffold-associated chondrocyte implantation

These so-called "second-generation autologous cartilage transplantation" techniques use biodegradable scaffolds to temporarily support the chondrocytes until they are replaced by matrix components synthesized from the implanted cells. Scaffolds can be based on carbohydrates (polylactic/polyglycolic acid, hyaluronan, agarose, alginate), protein polymers (collagen, fibrin, gelatin), artificial polymers (carbon fiber, hydroxyapatite, Teflon, polybutyric acid), or composite polymer matrices. Matrix-associated chondrocyte implantation (MACI) has been used with promising results in Europe and Australia but is not routinely available in the United States. The use of the biomatrix seeded with chondrocytes reduces surgical invasiveness and has the theoretic advantages of less chondrocyte leakage, more homogeneous chondrocyte distribution, and less graft hypertrophy. Ossendorf reported on 40 patients who underwent MACI with a polyglactin/polydiaxanone matrix scaffold,[68] Cincinnati, Lysholm, Knee injury and Osteoarthritis Outcome Score (KOOS), and SF-36 knee scores showed significant improvement at a 2-year follow-up. Biopsy at 12 months showed evidence of hyaline-like tissue, and MRI showed good defect filling. Bartlett compared porcine collagen membrane-ACI to porcine collagen biomatrix-ACI.[69] Both groups showed improvement in Cincinnati knee scores at 1 year with comparable amounts of hyaline cartilage and graft hypertrophy. Arthroscopic MACI has been described with a hyaluronic acid-based scaffold (Hyalograft-C, Fidia Advanced Biomaterials, Bologna, Italy) in 70 patients and showed improvement of knee function in 90%.[70] Better results were seen in patients younger than 30 years and athletes participating in higher-level competitive sports. Future developments are aimed at improving cellular matrix production by using more sophisticated bioactive scaffolds, which include growth factors and stimulate a more natural spatial distribution of chondrocytes within the repair cartilage.[71]

Cartilage autograft implantation

A different approach for autologous chondrocyte transplantation has been recently described, which provides delivery of autologous cartilage cells without ex vivo chondrocyte culture and expansion. In this technique, healthy cartilage tissue is harvested from

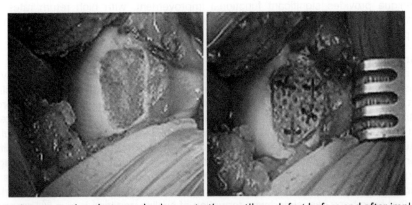

Fig. 3. Intraoperative photographs demonstrating cartilage defect before and after implantation of the Cartilage Autograft Implantation System (CAIS). (*Courtesy of* J. Farr, MD, Indianapolis, IN.)

an unaffected area of the injured joint and mechanically fragmented. The cartilage fragments are then embedded into a 3-D polymeric resorbable scaffold, which is then implanted into the auricular cartilage defect (Cartilage Autograft Implantation System (CAIS), J&J Regeneration Technologies, Raynham, MA) (**Fig. 3**). Experimental studies have demonstrated that outgrowth and migration of chondrocytes from the implanted cartilage fragments result in chondrocyte redistribution within the scaffold and produce hyaline-like repair tissue at 6 months.[72] This technique provides a single-stage procedure that avoids the complex and costly requirements of cell expansion. Clinical studies have shown the safety of this procedure and randomized, multi-center studies are currently under way to evaluate the clinical efficiency of this approach.

Neocartilage Implantation

Neocartilage implantation uses an advanced tissue engineering technology that generates an implant containing both chondrocytes and extracellular matrix.[73] With this

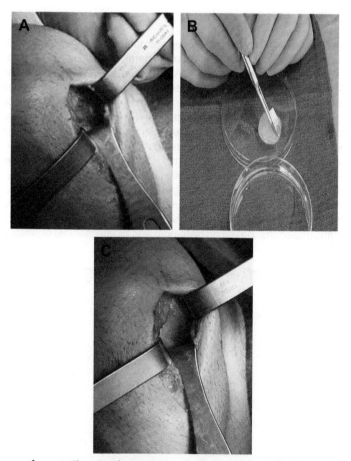

Fig. 4. Process of neocartilage implantation in a patient with an isolated chondral defect of the femoral condyle. Exposure and debridement of the defect can be done through miniarthrotomy (*A*), preparation of the neocartilage implant (NeoCart, Histogenics, Waltham, MA) (*B*), and appearance of the defect after implantation (*C*). (*Courtesy of* D. Crawford, MD, Portland, OR.)

two-step technique, autologous chondrocytes are extracted from harvested articular cartilage, expanded in a 2- D culture, and then seeded in a bovine collagen gel/sponge construct. Dynamic incubation of this 3-D construct under defined hydrostatic pressure in a specifically designed bioreactor stimulates the chondrocytes to produce cartilage matrix proteins, resulting in the formation of a firm sponge-like neocartilage containing both active chondrocytes and extracellular matrix (NeoCart, Histogenics, Waltham, MA).[74] Implantation is performed using a novel bioadhesive, which facilitates a minimally invasive surgical approach (**Fig. 4**). Because it bypasses the initial phase of chondrocyte implantation and in vivo matrix production, this technique may allow for shortening of the prolonged rehabilitation after cartilage repair and possibly earlier return to sport. Phase I trials showed good cartilage fill, peripheral integration, and pain relief in 86% up to 2 years after implantation (**Fig. 5**). Advanced MRI with T_2 mapping demonstrated tissue with signal characteristics similar to hyaline cartilage in 57% (**Fig. 6**). A larger prospective, randomized comparison of this technique with microfracture is currently being completed.

GENE THERAPY AND STEM CELLS

Gene therapy in combination with advanced tissue engineering methods offers some powerful options for enhancing articular cartilage repair and regeneration. Adenoviral-mediated transfection of cDNA encoding for TGF-β1, insulin-like growth factor 1 (IGF-I), BMP-7, and BMP-2 has been shown to stimulate expression of cartilage-specific extracellular matrix components and decreased chondrocyte dedifferentiation.[75] Genes can be transferred either into mature chondrocytes or into chondroprogenitor cells used for cartilage repair or regeneration. Pluripotent progenitor stem cells seem to be more receptive to transduction with recombinant adenoviral vectors and may provide the preferred platform for delivery of genes to enhance cartilage repair. Specifically, mesenchymal stem cells (MSC), found in bone marrow, skin, and adipose tissue, are capable of differentiating into articular cartilage as well as other cells of mesenchymal origin.[76] Hui and colleagues compared MSC transplants to cultured chondrocytes, osteochondral autograft, and periosteal grafts in animal models of osteochondritis dissecans. Based on histologic and biomechanical evaluation, several

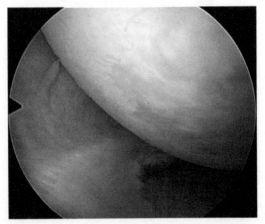

Fig. 5. Intraoperative photograph during unrelated meniscal surgery demonstrating flush appearance and complete peripheral integration of the neocartilage implant (NeoCart, Histogenics, Waltham, MA) 3 mo after implantation. (*Courtesy of* D. Crawford, MD, Portland, OR.)

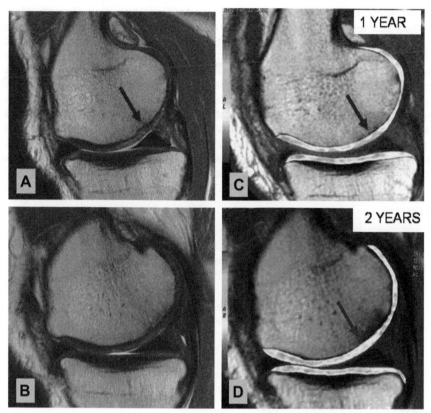

Fig. 6. Sagittal fast-spin-echo magnetic resonance image (*A, B*) and T$_2$ relaxation time mapping (*C, D*) of the knee 1 and 2 y following neocartilage implantation demonstrates complete fill of the defect, with full peripheral integration and improving tissue quality over time. (*Courtesy of* D. Crawford, MD, Portland, OR.)

studies found the MSC transplants to be comparable or superior to cultured chondrocytes and superior to periosteum and osteochondral autograft in their ability to repair chondral defects.[76,77,78] Stem cells alone or genetically modified MSC can be used to augment existing cell-based cartilage repair methods. MSCs derived from adipose tissue alone or transfected with a vector for BMP-2 have been shown to predictably heal cartilage defects, with increased hyaline cartilage quality by genetic engineering.[79,80] Experimental studies using implantation of polyglycolic acid scaffolds seeded with retrovirally transduced periosteal MSC expressing BMP-7 and sonic hedgehog (Shh) genes into osteochondral defects significantly enhanced the quality of the cartilage repair tissue, resulting in much smoother cartilage surfaces and increased hyaline morphology.[81] Although these techniques hold great scientific promise, they have not been confirmed in clinical studies but will very likely emerge as an option for treating cartilage injuries in athletes in the near future.

SUMMARY

Articular cartilage Injury in high-impact athletes has traditionally been associated with marked limitation of athletic activity and career-ending potential. The goal of articular cartilage restoration in this population is to return the athlete to pre-injury athletic participation and to minimize the potential for arthritic degeneration. Recently developed surgical techniques have shown that articular cartilage repair in this demanding population can successfully improve joint function and facilitate return to high-impact sports. The rate of improvement and ability to return to athletic activity is dependent on several factors, and the choice of repair technique should be tailored to individual patient and lesion characteristics. Each of the currently available repair techniques has been associated with specific limitations in terms of associated morbidity, repair tissue quality and quantity, clinical success rate, and durability of the functional improvement. Several novel scientific approaches are emerging that hold much promise to improve the current shortcomings and to produce an even higher-quality articular cartilage restoration, which permits superior ability to return to sport and minimizes the risk for secondary joint degeneration under continued athletic joint loading.

REFERENCES

1. Levy AS, Lohnes J, Sculley S, et al. Chondral delamination of the knee in soccer players. Am J Sports Med 1996;24:634–9.
2. Arendt E, Dick R. Knee injury patterns among men and women in collegiate basketball and soccer. NCAA data and review of literature. Am J Sports Med 1995;23:694–701.
3. Jones SJ, Lyons RA, Sibert J, et al. Changes in sports injuries to children between 1983 and 1998: comparison of case series. J Public Health Med 2001;23:268–71.
4. Moti AW, Micheli LJ. Meniscal and articular cartilage injury in the skeletally immature knee. Instr Course Lect 2003;52:683–90.
5. Smith AD, Tao SS. Knee injuries in young athletes. Clin Sports Med 1995;14:629–50.
6. Mandelbaum BT, Browne JE, Fu F, et al. Articular cartilage lesions of the knee. Am J Sports Med 2000;26:853–61.
7. Piasecki DD, Spindler KP, Warren TA, et al. Intraarticular injuries associated with anterior cruciate ligament tear: findings at ligament reconstruction in high school and recreational athletes. Am J Sports Med 2003;31:601–5.
8. Felson DT. Osteoarthritis: new insights. Part 1: the disease and its risk factors. Ann Intern Med 2000;133:635–46.
9. Kujala UM, Kettunen J, Paananen H, et al. Knee osteoarthritis in former runners, soccer players, weight lifters, and shooters. Arthritis Rheum 1995;38:539–46.
10. Jackson DW, Lalor PA, Aberman HM, et al. Spontaneous repair of full-thickness defects of articular cartilage in a goat model. J Bone Joint Surg Am 2001;83:53–64.
11. Buckwalter JA, Mankin HJ. Articular cartilage. Part II: degeneration and osteoarthrosis, repair, regeneration, and transplantation. J Bone Joint Surg Am 1997;79:612–32.
12. Vrahas MS, Mithoefer K, Joseph D. Long-term effects of articular impaction. Clin Orthop Rel Res 2004;423:40–3.
13. Lohmander LS, Roos H, Dahlberg L, et al. Temporal patterns of stromelysin, tissue inhibitor and proteoglycan fragments in synovial fluid after injury to the knee cruciate ligament or meniscus. J Orthop Res 1994;12:21–8.
14. Maletius W, Messner K. The long-term prognosis for severe damage to the weightbearing cartilage in the knee: a 14-year clinical and radiographic follow-up in 28 young athletes. Acta Orthop Scand 1996;165–8.
15. Hefti F, Beguiristain J, Krauspe R, et al. Osteochondritis dissecans: a multicenter study of the European pediatric orthopedic society. J Pediatr Orthop B 1999;8:231–45.

16. Drongowski RA, Coran AG, Woitys EM. Predictive value of meniscal and chondral injuries in conservatively treated anterior cruciate ligament injuries. Arthropscopy 1994;10:97–102.

17. Shelbourne KD, Jari S, Gray T. Outcome of untreated traumatic articular cartilage defects of the knee: a natural history study. J Bone Joint Surg Am 2003;85(Suppl 2): 8–16.

18. Drawer S, Fuller CW. Propensity for osteoarthritis and lower limb joint pain in retired professional soccer players. Br J Sports Med 2001;35:402–8.

19. Engstrom B, Forssblad M, Johansson C, et al. Does a major knee injury definitely sideline an elite soccer player? Am J Sports Med 1990;18:101–5.

20. Roos H. Are there long-term sequelae from soccer? Clin Sports Med 1998;17: 819–83.

21. Roos H, Lindberg H, Ornell M. Soccer as a cause of hip and knee osteoarthritis. Ann Rheum Dis 1996;55:690–8.

22. Jones G, Bennell K, Cicuttini FM. Effect of physical activity on cartilage development in healthy kids. Br J Sports Med 2003;37:382–3.

23. Kiviranta I, Tammi M, Jurvelin J. Articular cartilage thickness and glycosaminoglycan distribution in the canine knee joint after strenuous running exercise. Clin Orthop Rel Res 1992;283:302–8.

24. Arokoski J, Kiviranta I, Jurvelin J, et al. Long-distance running causes site-dependent decrease of cartilage glycosaminoglycan content in the knee joint of beagle dogs. Arthritis Rheum 1993;36:1451–9.

25. Buckwalter JA. Evaluating Methods for restoring cartilaginous articular surfaces. Clin Orthop Rel Res 1999;367S:S224–38.

26. Brittberg M, Lindahl A, Nilsson A, et al. Treatment of deep cartilage defects in the knee with autologous chondrocyte transplantation. N Engl J Med 1994;331: 889–95.

27. Steadman JR, Rodkey WG, Singleton SB, et al. Microfracture technique for full thickness chondral defects: technique and clinical results. Oper Tech Orthopedics 1997;7:300–4.

28. Hangody L, Rathonyi GK, Duska Z, Vasarhelyi G, et al. Autologous osteochondral mosaicplasty. Surgical technique. J Bone Joint Surg Am 2004;86(Suppl 1):65–72.

29. Gross A. Fresh osteochondral allograft for posttraumatic knee defects: Surgical technique. Op Tech Orthop 1997;7:334–9.

30. Jakobsen RB, Engebretsen L, Slauterbeck JR. An analysis of the quality of cartilage repair studies. J Bone Joint Surg Am 2005;87:2232–9.

31. Knutsen G, Drogset JO, Engebretsen L, et al. A randomized trial comparing autologous chondrocyte implantation with microfracture. J Bone Joint Surg Am 2008;90(5):1165–6.

32. Frisbee DD, Trotter GW, Powers BE, et al. Arthroscopic subchondral bone plate microfracture technique augments healing of large chondral defects in the radial carpal bone and medial femoral condyle of horses. Vet Surg 1999;28: 242–55.

33. Frisbie DD, Oxford JT, Southwood L, et al. Early events in cartilage repair after subchondral bone microfracture. Clin Orthop 2003;407:2115–227.

34. Gobbi A, Nunag P, Malinowski K. Treatment of chondral lesions of the knee with microfracture in a group of athletes. Knee Surg Sports Traumatol Arthrosc 2005; 13:213–21.

35. Steadman JR, Miller BS, Karas SG, et al. The microfracture technique in the treatment of full-thickness chondral lesions of the knee in national football league players. J Knee Surg 2003;16:83–6.

36. Blevins FT, Steadman JR, Rodrigo JJ, et al. Treatment of articular cartilage defects in athletes: an analysis of functional outcome and lesion appearance. Orthopedics 1998;21:761–8.
37. Mithoefer K, Williams RJ, Warren RF, et al. High-Impact athletics after knee articular cartilage repair. A prospective evaluation of the microfracture technique. Am J Sports Med 2006;34(9):1413–8.
38. Mithoefer K, Williams RJ, Warren RF, et al. The microfracture technique for treatment of articular cartilage lesions in the knee: a prospective cohort evaluation. J Bone Joint Surg 2005;87:1911–20.
39. Brown WE, Potter HG, Marx RG, et al. Magnetic resonance imaging appearance of cartilage repair in the knee. Clin Orthop 2004;422:214–23.
40. Neumann K, Dehne T, Endres, Erggelet C, et al. Chondrogenic differentiation capacity of human mesenchymal progenitor cells derived from subchondral corticospongious bone. J Orthop Res 2008;26(11):1449–56.
41. Kuo AC, Rodrigo JJ, Ah Reddi, ot al. Microfracture and bone morphogenetic protein 7 (BMP-7) synergistically stimulate articular cartilage repair. Ostooarthritis Cartil 2006;14:1126–35.
42. Morisset S, Frisbee DD, Robbins Pd, et al. Il-1ra/IGF-1 gene therapy modulates repair of microfractured chondral defects. Clin Orthop Rel Res 2007;462:221–8.
43. Hoemann CD, Hurtig M, Rossomacha E, et al. Chitosan-glycerol phosphate/blood implants improve hyaline cartilage repair in ovine microfracture defects. J Bone Joint Surg 2005;87:2671–86.
44. Wang DA, Varghese S, Sharma B, et al. Multifunctional chondroitin sulphate for cartilage tissue-biomaterial integration. Nat Mater 2007;6(5):385–92.
45. Hoemann CD, Sun J, McKee MD, et al. Chitosan-glycerol phosphate/blood implants elicit hyaline cartilage repair integrated with porous subchondral bone in microdrilled rabbit defects. Osteoarthritis Cartilage 2007;15:78–89.
46. Buschmann MD, Hoemann CD, Hurtig MB, et al. Cartilage repair with chitosan-glycerol phosphate stabilized blood clots. In: Williams RJ, editor. Cartilage repair strategies. Totawa (NJ): Humana press; 2007. p. 85–104.
47. Hangody L, Fule P. Autologous osteochondral mosaicplasty for the treatment of full thickness defects of weight bearing joints: ten years of experimental and clinical experience. J Bone Joint Surg Am 2003;85(Suppl 2):25–32.
48. Kish G, Modis L, Hangody L. Osteochondral mosaicplasty for the treatment of focal chondral and osteochondral lesions of the knee and talus in the athlete. Rationale, indications, technique, and results. Clin Sports Med 1999;18:45–66.
49. Gudas R, Kelesinskas RJ, Kimtys V, et al. A prospective randomized clinical study of mosaic osteochondral autologous transplantation versus microfracture for the treatment of osteochondral defects in the knee joint in young athletes. Arthroscopy 2005;21:1066–75.
50. Whiteside RA, Bryant JT, Jakob RP, et al. Short-term load bearing capacity of osteochondral autografts implanted by the mosaicplasty technique: an in vitro porcine model. J Biomech 2003;36:1203–8.
51. Koh J, Wirsing K, Lautenschlager E, et al. The effect of graft height mismatch on contact pressures following osteochondral grafting. Am J Sports Med 2004;32:317–20.
52. Horas U, Pelinkovic D, Aigner T. Autologous chondrocyte implantation and osteochondral cylinder transplantation in cartilage repair of the knee joint: a prospective comparative trial. J Bone Joint Surg Am 2003;85:185–92.
53. Huntley J, Bush P, McBurnie J. Chondrocyte death associated with human femoral osteochondral harvest as performed for mosaicplasty. J Bone Joint Surg Am 2005;87:351–60.

54. LaPrade RF, Botker JC. Donor-site morbidity after osteochondral autograft transfer procedures. Arthroscopy 2004;20:e69–73.
55. Williams RJ, Dreese JC, Chen CT. Chondrocyte survival and material properties of hypothermically stored cartilage: an evaluation of tissue used for osteochondral allograft transplantation. Am J Sports Med 2004;32:132–9.
56. Gross AE, Shahsa N, Aubin P. Long-term followup of the fresh osteochondral allografts for posttraumatic knee defects. Clin Orthop Relat Res 2005;435:79–87.
57. Shasha N, Aubin PP, Cheah HK, et al. Long-term clinical experience with fresh osteochondral allografts for articular knee defects in high-demand patients. Cell Tissue Bank 2002;3:175–82.
58. Williams RJ, Gamrath SC. Articular cartilage repair using a resorbable matrix scaffold. Instr Course Lect 2008;57:563–71.
59. Williams RJ, Niederauer GG. Articular cartilage resurfacing using synthetic resorbable scaffolds. In: Williams RJ, editor. Cartilage repair strategies. Totawa (NJ): Humana press; 2007. p. 115–36.
60. Peterson L, Minas T, Brittberg M, et al. Two- to 9-year outcome after autologous chondrocyte transplantation of the knee. Clin Orthop Rel Res 2000;374:212–34.
61. Peterson L, Brittberg M, Kiviranta I, et al. Autologous chondrocyte transplantation. Biomechanics and long-term durability. Am J Sports Med 2002;30:2–12.
62. Knutsen G, Engebretsen L, Ludvigsen TC, et al. Autologous chondrocyte transplantation compared with microfracture in the knee. A randomized trial. J Bone Joint Surg Am 2004;86:455–64.
63. Mithöfer K, Peterson L, Mandelbaum BR, et al. Articular cartilage repair in soccer players with autologous chondrocyte transplantation: Functional outcome and return to competition. Am J Sports Med 2005;33(11):1639–46.
64. Mithöfer K, Minas T, Peterson L, et al. Functional outcome of articular cartilage repair in adolescent athletes. Am J Sports Med 2005;33:1147–53.
65. Kreuz PC, Steinwachs M, Erggelet C, et al. Importance of sports in cartilage regeneration after autologous chondrocyte implantation. Am J Sports Med 2007;35:1261–8.
66. Saris DBF, Vanlauwe J, Victor J, et al. Characterized chondrocyte implantation results in better structural repair when treating symptomatic cartilage defects of the knee in a randomized controlled trial versus microfracture. Am J Sports Med 2008;36(2):235–46.
67. Dell'Accio F, De Bari C, Luyten FP. Molecular markers predictive of the capacity of expanded human articular chondrocytes to form stable cartilage in vivo. Arthritis Rheum 2001;44(7):1608–19.
68. Ossendorf C, Kaps C, Kreuz PC, et al. Treatment of posttraumatic and focal osteoarthritic cartilage defects of the knee with autologous polymer-based three-dimensional chondrocyte grafts: 2-year clinical results. Arthritis Res Ther 2007;9(2):640–5.
69. Bartlett W, Skinner JA, Gooding CR, et al. Autologous chondrocyte implantation versus matrix-induced autologous chondrocyte implantation for osteochondral defects of the knee: a prospective, randomized study. J Bone Joint Surg Br 2005;87:640–5.
70. Marcacci M, Kon E, Delcogliano M, et al. Arthroscopic autologous osteochondral grafting for cartilage defects of the knee: prospective study results at a minimum 7-year follow-up. Am J Sports Med 2007;35(12):2014–21.
71. Chou CH, Cheng WT, Lin CC, et al. TGF-beta1 immobilized tri-co-polymer for articular cartilage tissue engineering. J Biomed Mater Res B Appl Biomater 2006;77(2):338–48.

72. Lu Y, Dhanaraj S, Wang Z, et al. Minced cartilage without cell culture serves as an effective intraoperative cell source for cartilage repair. J Orthop Res 2006;24:1261–70.
73. Kim HT, Zaffagini S, Mizuno S, et al. A peek into the possible future of management of articular cartilage injuries: gene therapy and scaffolds for cartilage repair. J Orthop Sports Phys Ther 2006;36:765–73.
74. Mizuno S, Tateishi T, Ushida T, et al Hydrostatic fluid pressure enhances matrix synthesis and accumulation by bovine chondrocytes in three-dimensional culture. J Cell Physiol 2002;193:319–27.
75. Steinert AF, Palmer GD, Ghivizzani SC, et al. Gene therapy in the treatment of cartilage injury. In: Mirzayan R, editor. Cartilage injury in the athlete. New York: Thieme; 2006 p. 297–308.
76. Liu Y, Shu XZ, Prestwich GD. Osteochondral defect repair with autologous bone marrow-derived mesenchymal stem cells in an injectable, in situ, cross-linked synthetic extracellular matrix. Tissue Eng 2006;12:3405–16.
77. Yan H, Yu C. Repair of full-thickness cartilage defects with cells of different origin in a rabbit model. Arthroscopy 2007;23:178–87.
78. Hui JH, Chen F, Thambyah A, et al. Treatment of chondral lesions in advanced osteochondritis dissecans: a comparative study of the efficacy of chondrocytes, mesenchymal stem cells, periosteal graft, and mosaicplasty (osteochondral autograft) in animal models. J Pediatri Orthop 2004;24:427–33.
79. Dragoo JL, Carlson G, McCormick F, et al. Healing full-thickness cartilage defects using adipose-derived stem cells. Tissue Engineering 2007;13:1–7.
80. Dragoo JL, Samimi B, Zhu M, et al. Tissue-engineered cartilage and bone using stem cells from human infrapatellar fat pads. J Bone Joint Surg Br 2003;85B: 740–7.
81. Grande DA, Mason J, Light E, et al. Stem cells as platforms for delivery of genes to enhance cartilage repair. JBJS Am 2003;85:111–6.

Surgical Navigation in Knee Ligament Reconstruction

D. Kendoff, MD, PhD*, M. Citak, MD, J. Voos, MD, A.D. Pearle, MD

KEYWORDS

- Navigation • ACL reconstruction • Computer-assisted surgery
- Knee stability • PCL • MCL

The number of anterior cruciate ligament (ACL) reconstructions in the United States continues to increase, with over 100,000 primary reconstructions currently performed each year.[1] The single incision, endoscopic transtibial tunnel technique is used most often. Visual identification of femoral and tibial tunnel placements is based on arthroscopic landmarks and conventions. The revision rate ranges from 10% to 40%, of which 70% to 80% of the complications are due to malpositioned tunnels.[2] Although the overall outcome of ACL reconstruction is successful in up to 90% of patients, some high-level athletes may complain of continued feelings of instability and subsequent decreased productivity.

Several studies have shown non-physiologic dynamic knee kinematics after ACL reconstruction. Logan and colleagues[3] showed that the amount of excursion between the tibial and femoral joint surfaces was similar between the normal and reconstructed knees, but the relationship of tibia to femur was always different for each position of knee flexion assessed. The lateral tibia was 5 mm more anterior in the ACL-reconstructed knees. They concluded that ACL reconstruction reduces sagittal laxity to within normal limits but does not restore normal tibiofemoral kinematics despite a successful outcome. Tashman and colleagues[4] also showed that abnormal rotational knee motion occurred and failed to restore normal knee kinematics after reconstruction. Another study by Chouliaras and colleagues[5] found significantly increased tibial rotation compared with a control group. Taken together, these studies demonstrate that current techniques for ACL reconstruction fail to restore normal knee kinematics. Based on these results and other clinical and laboratory research, computer navigation has been employed in an attempt to improve clinical outcomes by standardizing tunnel placement and restoring knee kinematics closer to physiologic conditions after ACL reconstruction.

Sports Medicine and Shoulder Service, The Hospital for Special Surgery, New York, NY, USA
* Corresponding author. Department of Orthopaedic Surgery, Computer Assisted Surgery Center, Hospital for Special Surgery, 535 East, 70th Street, New York, NY 10021.
E-mail address: kendoffd@hss.edu (D. Kendoff).

Clin Sports Med 28 (2009) 41–50
doi:10.1016/j.csm.2008.08.010
0278-5919/08/$ – see front matter
sportsmed.theclinics.com

Historically, one of the first applications using modern navigation techniques in orthopedic surgery was ACL reconstruction.[6,7] The first described clinical, image-free navigated case for an ACL reconstruction was reported in 1995 by Dessenne and colleagues.[8] Further developments included the ability to assess the placement of femoral and tibial tunnels, ligament impingement, and isometric projections.[6,7,9–12] More recently, stability testing including rotational and translational measurements became possible with current navigation systems. This review provides an overview of the current applications and limitations of computer navigation in knee ligament reconstruction by reviewing the current available literature. A Medline search was performed of the terms "computer navigation," "surgical navigation," "ACL reconstruction," "PCL reconstruction," and "MCL reconstruction" to access all available articles on the topic.

ACL NAVIGATION OVERVIEW

Surgical navigation typically offers an augmented, 3D view of the surgical field to assist with decision making. In addition, navigation can provide quantitative feedback to help supervise surgical procedures. Navigation technologies are most compelling when clinically relevant surgical targets with defined tolerances have been established. As such, the use of surgical navigation for tunnel placement in ACL surgery remains inherently problematic because the optimal position for placement of ACL tunnels remains debatable. As such, there is no single ACL tunnel position that is ideal for navigation.

Various strategies to optimize tunnel positioning have been used in different commercially available navigation systems. The most common means of supervising tunnel placement include

- Isometry profile (length changes) during flexion/extension
- Impingement profiles of a virtual graft (**Fig. 1**)
- Anatomic landmarks (**Fig. 2**)
- Radiographic criteria (**Fig. 3**)

With isometry-based modules, a virtual graft is placed and the length changes are reported during a flexion/extension cycle. This allows the surgeon to modify graft position to optimize the isometry profile (Praxim, Grenoble, France) (see **Fig. 1**). Impingement conflicts are reported in some modules, alerting the surgeon to potential areas were a graft may impinge. Arthroscopic anatomic landmarks, which are surgeon defined, can be used to quantify graft position in relation to the clock face in the notch and the spines on the tibia (Orthopilot, Tuttlingen, Germany). Finally, systems can use radiographic landmarks and measurements using fluoroscopic imaging to guide tunnel placement (Brainlab, Feldkirchen, Germany) (see **Fig. 3**). Current systems often offer combinations of these criteria in an "a la carte" menu.

In addition to supervising tunnel position, current systems offer a means to quantify stability examination before and after reconstruction. While navigation systems have been shown to be accurate in tracking motions, application of standard loads during navigated stability examination remains problematic.

REVIEW OF CURRENT LITERATURE

The number of navigated ACL reconstructions has grown rapidly in recent years (**Table 1**).[13] Before 2006 only 9 Medline listed publications referring to "navigation" and "ACL reconstructions" could be found. As of May 2008, the search revealed 32 publications. Initial reports focused primarily on the feasibility of computer navigation

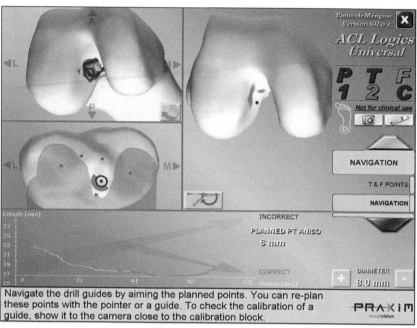

Fig. 1. Intraoperative navigated screenshot of ACL reconstruction allowing optimization of tunnel placements based on the isometry of a virtually placed graft (Praxim, Grenoble, France).

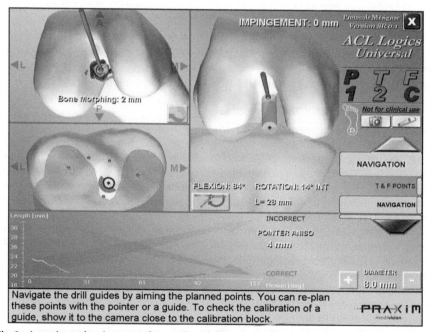

Fig. 2. A navigated pointer can be used to define optimal femoral and tibial tunnel placement, thus simulating eventual graft impingement throughout the complete knee motion path. The isometry of the virtual graft can also be visualized (Praxim, Grenoble, France).

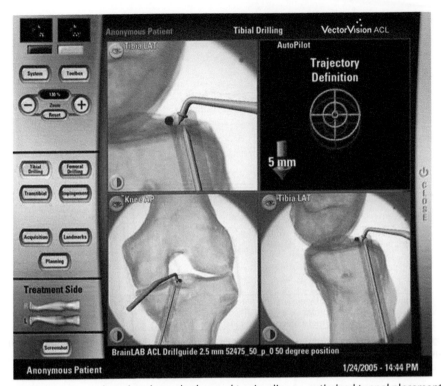

Fig. 3. A fluoroscopy-based tool can also be used to visualize an optimized tunnel placement in multiple radiographic planes (BrainLAB, Feldkirchen, Germany).

for ACL reconstruction or laboratory testing.[6–8] Recent publications have focused on either prospective or retrospective measurements of clinical outcome parameters comparing navigated and conventional ACL reconstruction techniques.[6,7,9–12]

Navigated Tunnel Placement

Dessenne and colleagues[8] reported in 1995 that computer-based navigation techniques had been successfully tested in primary ACL reconstructions in 12 patients. Jalliard and colleagues[7] in 1998 concluded in a cadaveric study that computer navigation techniques made it possible to assess graft configurations that avoid notch impingement. Bernsmann and colleagues[6] concluded that navigation is able to give the surgeon views that are not achieved with conventional surgery. The feasibility of this device in routine clinical use has been proven.

In 1998, Klos and colleagues[9] compared conventional tunnel placement to fluoroscopic visualization with computer overlays. They found significant reduction in graft placement variability from radiographic assessment of tunnel placement in the tibia and femur in the fluoroscopy and computer-assistance group compared with the conventional tunnel placement group. This study concluded that simple visual enhancements seem to be useful in improving the repeatability of arthroscopic ACL reconstruction using radiographic measurements as the outcome parameter.

In a randomized laboratory study by Picard and colleagues[11] using a foam knee model and an image-based navigation device, it was reported that the accuracy of tunnel placement with navigation was significantly better than that obtained with the

Table 1
Summary of Medline-listed publications including "navigation" and "ACL reconstruction" before and after 2006

Author	Year	Study Type	Tunnel Placement	Kinematics
Ishibashi et al.	2008	Review		X
Kodali et al.	2008	Review	X	X
Hart et al.	2008	Clinical	X	
Zaffagnini et al.	2008	Laboratory	X	X
Tsukada et al.	2008	Laboratory	X	
Pearle et al.	2008	Laboratory	X	
Lane et al.	2008	Clinical		X
Seon et al.	2008	Clinical		X
Martelli et al.	2008	Clinical		X
Tsuda et al.	2007	Laboratory	X	
Monaco et al.	2007	Clinical		X
Martelli et al.	2007	Clinical		X
Hart et al.	2007	Review	X	X
Kendoff et al.	2007	Laboratory		X
Nakagawa et al.	2007	Technical Note	X	
Zhang et al.	2007	Clinical	X	
Tanaka et al.	2007	Laboratory		X
Colombet et al.	2007	Laboratory		X
Panisset et al.	2006	Clinical	X	
Koh et al.	2006	Clinical	X	
Ishibashi et al.	2006	Laboratory	X	
Hiraoka et al.	2006	Clinical	X	
Martelli et al.	2006	Laboratory		X
Author et al.	Year	Study Type	Tunnel Placement	Kinematics
Koh	2005	Review	X	X
Ishibashi et al.	2005	Clinical		X
Schep et al.	2005	Laboratory	X	
Degenhart et al.	2005	Unknown	X	
Liao et al.	2005	Clinical	X	
Mueller-Alsbach et al.	2004	Technical Description	X	
Sabczynshi et al.	2004	Unknown	X	
Picard et al.	2001	Laboratory	X	
Bernsmann et al.	2001	Clinical	X	

traditional arthroscopic techniques. Distances from the ideal tunnel placement to the femoral and tibial tunnels were statistically better in the group using navigation. Distances to ideal tibial and femoral tunnel placements were 4.2 ± 1.8 mm and 4.9 ± 2.3 mm, respectively, for the standard technique and 2.7 ± 1.9 mm and 3.4 ± 2.3 mm for the navigated group, respectively. Hiraoka and colleagues,[14] using a fluoroscopy-based module, found that navigation improves accuracy and decreases dispersion of the tibial tunnel placement in single-bundle ACL reconstruction compared with an endoscopic technique.

Another laboratory study by Schep and colleagues[15] found that computer-assisted planning of ACL tunnel positions reduces surgical variance and elongation or impingement of virtual grafts compared with a conventional arthroscopic technique. Muller-Alsbach and colleagues[16] reported assessing the placement of a virtual graft and corresponding tunnel with computer navigation before real graft implantation might reduce the risks for notch impingement. However, their study did not include any clinical data.

In a randomized, controlled trial, Mauch and colleagues[10] reported clinical outcomes in 53 athletes randomized to conventional ACL reconstruction versus computer-assisted ACL reconstruction. Outcomes were focused on tibial tunnel placement by evaluating lateral radiographs. The results of this study showed no significant difference in the location and variability of the tibial tunnel placement when comparing both groups. However, significant differences were found when the center of the tibial tunnels for both groups was compared with the ideal tibial tunnel placement reported in the literature. The study concluded that computer-assisted navigation offers good support for correct placement of the tibial tunnel, although experienced surgeons can achieve the same positioning as surgeons using computer-assisted navigation.

Navigated Knee Stability Examination

In addition to facilitating tunnel placement, navigation also provides the ability to assess ligament stability and tibio-femoral translations and rotations. The ability to accurately measure ligament integrity allows flexibility in intraoperative and postoperative assessment of knee kinematics. In a cadaver model, Kendoff and colleagues[17] compared navigated measurements of tibial anteroposterior (AP) translation and rotation with mechanical measuring devices: the KT 1000 and a modified goniometer tool. Tests were repeated with intact and ACL-deficient specimens, and measurements of translation and rotation were statistically compared. There was no significant difference in AP translation and tibial rotation between computer navigation and KT 1000 ($P > .05$). Tibial rotation revealed no significant difference between navigation and goniometer measurements ($P > .05$). This study concluded that stability parameters in ACL navigation can be measured precisely under laboratory conditions and results are not significantly different from mechanical testing devices.

Pearle and colleagues,[18] in a cadaveric model using a 6 degree of freedom robotic testing system, demonstrated a near-perfect correlation between an image-free navigation system and a robotic sensor in tracking coupled knee motions. Consequently, navigation systems can be used as a precise intraoperative multiplanar arthrometer and may help delineate pathologic multiplanar or coupled knee motions, particularly in the setting of complex rotatory instability patterns. However, application of standardized loads during stability testing remains challenging. In addition, accurate tracking of knee motion is predicated on rigid bony fixation of trackers, so comparative examinations of the contralateral limb are problematic.

Several authors have now reported computer-navigated stability examinations as a means of documenting the efficacy of navigated, double bundle, or other technical approaches to ACL reconstruction. Ishibashi and colleagues[19] presented a study of 32 patients undergoing double-bundle ACL reconstruction. AP displacement and rotation of the tibia were measured before reconstruction and after posterolateral bundle fixation, anteromedial (AM) bundle fixation, and double-bundle ACL reconstruction. Using navigated stability examinations, the authors demonstrated that the posterolateral bundle has an important role in the extension position, whereas the AM bundle restricts AP displacement from extension to flexion. AP displacement after double-bundle ACL reconstruction was significantly improved compared with AP displacement after posterolateral-bundle or AM bundle fixation. Colombet and colleagues[20] reported comparable results using tibiofemoral rotation kinematics before and after ACL reconstruction.

Koh[21] quantified in vivo translation and rotational stability preoperatively and postoperatively in 52 patients undergoing ACL reconstruction using computer navigation. Translation was calculated by the computer while performing a Lachman maneuver. Medial and lateral rotations were calculated by the computer and the final outcome measure was a total arc of rotation that equaled the sum of medial and lateral rotations. Anterior translation was significantly decreased after reconstruction ($P<.005$). A significant decrease ($P<.005$) in arc of rotation was also noted after ACL reconstruction. These studies provide quantitative time zero benchmarks for multiplanar motions during stability examination before and after various ACL reconstruction strategies. The relationship between time zero measurements and long-term outcomes is unclear.

In addition to uniplanar, AP translation tests such as the Lachman and anterior drawer, rotational maneuvers, including the pivot-shift examination, are possible using navigation systems. Lane and colleagues[22] recently reported retrospectively on 12 patients who underwent navigated ACL surgery. A navigated pivot-shift examination was performed and correlated with clinical grading of the maneuver. A characteristic P-shaped track of motion was recorded by the navigation software during the pivot-shift examination. The "angle of P" was developed as a means of characterizing this track of motion and was measured in all cases. It was concluded that clinical quantification of the distinct elements of the pivot shift may allow for more accurate evaluation of different ACL reconstruction constructs. There is also potential for these variables to be measured intraoperatively and to guide ACL reconstruction.

Clinical Outcomes of Navigated Versus Conventional ACL Reconstruction

Plaweski and colleagues[12] presented a randomized, controlled clinical trial of ACL reconstructions in 60 patients, in which 30 patients underwent conventional ACL reconstruction and 30 patients underwent surgery using computer navigation. Outcomes were assessed with dynamic stress radiographs to measure laxity at 150 and 200 N anterior loads and evaluation of radiographic tunnel positioning. There was no significant difference in absolute laxity, but a significant difference was noted in the variability of laxity ($P = .003$). At a 2-year follow up, 96.7% of patients in the navigated group had < 2-mm laxity at 150 N postoperative stress radiographic testing compared with 83% in the conventional group. Tibial tunnel placement was also significantly improved in the navigated group compared with the conventional group. Additionally, 23.3% of the conventional group had > 3 mm side-to-side difference in Lachman compared with 13% of the navigated group at 24 months follow-up. Similarly, 23.4% of the conventional group exhibited mild glide in the pivot-shift test in contrast to 13% mild pivot in the navigated group. This study confirms that the accuracy and consistency of tibial tunnel position can be improved by the use of computer-assisted navigation and that the clinical result in terms of laxity is more reliable.

On the other hand, a clinical comparative study by Hart[23] found no functionally important differences in 40 patients undergoing navigated versus 40 patients undergoing conventional ACL reconstructions. Although no relevant differences were found for postoperative functionality and AP laxity for both groups, radiographic differences were found for the femoral tunnel placements. Navigation allowed for a more accurate placement of the femoral tunnel, whereas it did not improve the tibial tunnel accuracy compared with the conventional technique.

The goal of surgical navigation is to use quantitative feedback to make surgery more precise, minimally invasive, and patient specific. This quantitative feedback is predicated on established targets and tolerances. This remains problematic in ACL surgery as targets for graft positioning and navigated stability examination remain poorly defined, especially when patient variables, such as notch anatomy, alignment, and generalized laxity, are considered. In a series of cadaveric studies, Pearle and colleagues[18] have defined normative 3-dimensional obliquity data for anatomic ACL fiber positions at various flexion angles and have defined how these fibers respond to different loading conditions. These normative data can be compared with intraoperative data and may allow for more refined graft position targeting. Indeed, based on these unique data generated with navigation, Pearle and colleagues recently demonstrated that the conventional ACL graft position using a transtibial approach is 10 to 15 degrees more vertical in both the coronal and sagittal plane at multiple flexion angles, which may provide an anatomic explanation for the failure of single-bundle ACL reconstruction to restore intact knee kinematics.

POSTERIOR CRUCIATE LIGAMENT NAVIGATION

There is currently no available clinical literature on posterior cruciate ligament (PCL) reconstructions using computer navigation. Navigation modules do exist that are able to measure the isometric profile and impingement conflicts of a virtually placed graft.

Existing laboratory studies have used computer-based calculations of 3-dimensional knee kinematic parameters and estimations of combined graft deformation after different PCL reconstruction techniques. These studies were able to show that computer-based simulation methods provided valid quantitative information concerning restoration of AP and rotational laxity as well as kinematic curves.[24,25]

MEDIAL COLLATERAL LIGAMENT NAVIGATION

Currently no scientific report on the use of navigation in medial collateral ligament (MCL) reconstruction has been found in a Medline search. Although some reports discuss the indirect influence of the MCL on navigated measurements of mechanical lower limb axis, no distinct use for MCL reconstruction exists to the authors' knowledge. Existing software modules include measurement of the specific MCL length during the flexion-extension arc, based on insertion landmarks defined by the bone surface registration technique with a navigated pointer. Based on the defined femoral insertion site, calculated isometric graft behavior can be visualized, to define the optimal tibial insertion (**Fig. 4**).

FUTURE APPLICATIONS

In addition to intraoperative assessment of tunnel placement and the ability to objectively measure knee stability before and after ACL reconstruction, future applications of computer navigation will allow measurement of knee kinematics pre- and postoperatively. Furthermore, a direct contralateral comparison to the "healthy," intact knee could provide relevant information about knee kinematics and stability. The limiting factor in establishing navigation as a conventional measurement tool in regular nonoperative use is the necessity for rigid fixation of the reference markers. Currently, only absolute rigid fixation using percutaneous cortical fixation during lower limb movements and kinematic evaluations can assure accurate navigated measurements. Although alternative fixation techniques have been introduced, no reproducible clinical use has been achieved to observe knee kinematics. Future innovations may allow for a soft-tissue reference marker fixation.

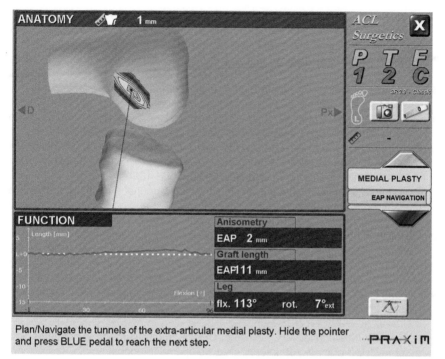

Fig. 4. Screenshot of a specific MCL length measurement during the flexion-extension arc. Based on the defined femoral insertion site, calculated isometric graft behavior can be visualized, to define the optimal tibial insertion (Praxim, Grenoble, France).

As the size and portability of computer navigation continue to improve, portable computer-based navigation and mini infrared camera systems may allow standardized use in the outpatient clinic. This would provide valuable quantification of knee stability pre-, intra-, and, finally, postoperatively after ACL and other ligament reconstructions while being compared with the contralateral intact knee.

As additional clinical studies are performed and technology improves, the clinical utility of computer navigation will continue to be defined.

REFERENCES

1. Bach BR Jr, Aadalen KJ, Dennis MG, et al. Primary anterior cruciate ligament reconstruction using fresh-frozen, nonirradiated patellar tendon allograft: minimum 2-year follow-up. Am J Sports Med 2005;33(2):284–92.
2. Wetzler M, Bartolozzi A, Gillespie M, et al. Revision anterior cruciate ligament reconstruction. Operative Techniques in Orthopaedics 1996;6:181–9.
3. Logan MC, Williams A, Lavelle J, et al. Tibiofemoral kinematics following successful anterior cruciate ligament reconstruction using dynamic multiple resonance imaging. Am J Sports Med 2004;32(4):984–92.
4. Tashman S, Kolowich P, Collon D, et al. Dynamic function of the ACL-reconstructed knee during running. Clin Orthop Relat Res 2007;454:66–73.
5. Chouliaras V, Ristanis S, Moraiti C, et al. Effectiveness of reconstruction of the anterior cruciate ligament with quadrupled hamstrings and bone-patellar tendon-bone autografts: an in vivo study comparing tibial internal-external rotation. Am J Sports Med 2007;35(2):189–96.

6. Bernsmann K, Rosenthal A, Sati M, et al. Using the CAS (computer-assisted surgery) system in arthroscopic cruciate ligament surgery–adaptation and application in clinical practice. Z Orthop Ihre Grenzgeb 2001;139(4):346–51.
7. Jalliard R, Lavallee S, Dessenne V. Computer assisted reconstruction of the anterior cruciate ligament. Clin Orthop Relat Res 1998;354:57–64.
8. Dessenne V, Lavallee S, Julliard R, et al. Computer-assisted knee anterior cruciate ligament reconstruction: first clinical tests. J Image Guid Surg 1995;1(1):59–64.
9. Klos T, Habets R, Banks A, et al. Computer assistance in arthroscopic anterior cruciate ligament reconstruction. Clin Orthop Relat Res 1998;354:65–9.
10. Mauch F, Apic G, Becker U, et al. Differences in the placement of the tibial tunnel during reconstruction of the anterior cruciate ligament with and without computer-assisted navigation. Am J Sports Med 2007;35(11):1824–32.
11. Picard F, DiGioia AM, Moody J, et al. Accuracy in tunnel placement for ACL reconstruction. Comparison of traditional arthroscopic and computer-assisted navigation techniques. Comput Aided Surg 2001;6(5):279–89
12. Plaweski S, Cazal J, Rosell P, et al. Anterior cruciate ligament reconstruction using navigation: a comparative study on 60 patients. Am J Sports Med 2006;34:542–52.
13. Valentin P, Hofbauer M, Aldrian S. Clinical results of computer-navigated anterior cruciate ligament reconstructions. Orthopedics 2005;28(Suppl 10):s1289–91.
14. Hiraoka H, Kuribayashi S, Fukuda A, et al. Endoscopic anterior cruciate ligament reconstruction using a computer-assisted fluoroscopic navigation system. J Orthop Sci 2006;11(2):159–66.
15. Schep NW, Stavenuiter MH, Diekerhof CH, et al. Intersurgeon variance in computer-assisted planning of anterior cruciate ligament reconstruction. Arthroscopy 2005;21(8):942–7.
16. Muller-Alsbach UW, Staubli AE. Computer aided ACL reconstruction. Injury 2004;35(Suppl 1):S-A65–7.
17. Kendoff D, Meller R, Citak M, et al. Navigation in ACL reconstruction - comparison with conventional measurement tools. Technol Health Care 2007;15(3):221–30.
18. Pearle AD, Shannon FJ, Granchi C, et al. Comparison of 3-dimensional obliquity and anisometric characteristics of anterior cruciateligament graft positions using surgical navigation. Am J Sports Med 2008;36(8):1534–41.
19. Ishibashi Y, Tsuda E, Tazawa K, et al. Intraoperative evaluation of the anatomical double-bundle anterior cruciate ligament reconstruction with the OrthoPilot navigation system. Orthopedics 2005;28(Suppl 10):s1277–82.
20. Colombet P, Robinson J, Christel P, et al. Using navigation to measure rotation kinematics during ACL reconstruction. Clin Orthop Relat Res 2007;454:59–65.
21. Koh J. Computer-assisted navigation and anterior cruciate ligament reconstruction: accuracy and outcomes. Orthopedics 2005;28(Suppl 10):s1283–7.
22. Lane CG, Warren RF, Stanford FC, et al. In vivo analysis of the pivot shift phenomenon during computer navigated ACL reconstruction. Knee Surg Sports Traumatol Arthrosc 2008, in press.
23. Hart R, Krejzla J, Sváb P, et al. Outcomes after conventional versus computer-navigated anterior cruciate ligament reconstruction. Arthroscopy 2008;24(5):569–78.
24. Boisgard S, Levai JP, Saidane K, et al. Study of the posterior cruciate ligament using a 3D computer model: ligament biometry during flexion, application to surgical replacement of the ligament. Acta Orthop Belg 1999;65(4):492–502.
25. Hagemeister N, Duval N, Yahia L, et al. Comparison of two methods for reconstruction of the posterior cruciate ligament using a computer based method: quantitative evaluation of laxity, three-dimensional kinematics and ligament deformation measurement in cadaver knees. Knee 2002;9(4):291–9.

Current Status and Potential of Primary ACL Repair

Martha M. Murray, MD

KEYWORDS

- Anterior cruciate ligament • Repair • Regeneration
- Collagen-platelet • Composite • Fibroblast

CLINICAL SIGNIFICANCE OF ACL INJURY

Ruptures of the ACL of the knee affect over 175,000 patients every year, including an estimated 38,000 high school students.[1] These injuries are devastating, not only at the time of the acute injury but also because patients who sustain an ACL tear have a 78% risk of radiographic osteoarthritis within 14 years following their injury (**Fig. 1**), whether they undergo surgical reconstruction or not.[2] For a high school or college student with an ACL tear, that is a striking and troubling statistic.

Current Treatment of ACL Tears

The ACL has long been thought to have poor capacity for healing, even with suture repair. Rates of failure of healing (non-union) and structural laxity of the ACL, even with surgical repair, range from 40% to 100%.[3–5] This is in contrast to other ligaments, such as the medial collateral ligament (MCL), where successful healing is essentially universally achievable with only 6 weeks of brace treatment. The lack of functional healing seen in the ACL after suture repair has been previously attributed to the "hostile" environment of synovial fluid,[6,7] to alterations in the cellular metabolism after injury,[8,9] and to intrinsic cell deficiencies.[10–16] This has led to abandonment of suture repair and almost universal adoption of ACL reconstruction for treatment. In ACL reconstruction, the torn ACL tissue is removed from the knee surgically and replaced with a tendon graft harvested from the medial hamstrings, the middle third of the patellar tendon, or allograft tissue.

However, although ACL reconstruction is an excellent operation for restoring the sagittal plane stability of the knee, significant problems remain. In the short term,

Martha Murray, author of "Current status and potential of primary repair of the ACL" has stock ownership and serves on the Scientific Advisory Board of Connective Orthopaedics. The article was written and accepted before this affiliation.
Department of Orthopaedic Surgery, Children's Hospital of Boston, Hunnewell 2, 300 Longwood Avenue, Boston, MA 02115, USA
E-mail address: martha.murray@childrens.harvard.edu

Clin Sports Med 28 (2009) 51–61
doi:10.1016/j.csm.2008.08.005
0278-5919/08/$ – see front matter © 2008 Elsevier Inc. All rights reserved.

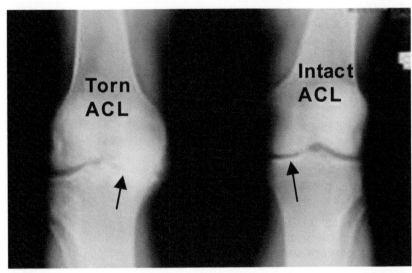

Fig.1. Premature osteoarthritis after ACL injury. Radiographs of a 40-year-old man who had sustained an ACL rupture 20 years earlier. Note the joint space narrowing and osteophyte formation consistent with premature osteoarthritis (*arrow*) on the medial aspect of the left knee (knee with ACL tear) and the preservation of medial joint space in the knee with the intact ACL on the right (*arrow*).

ACL reconstruction requires harvesting of other tissues from the knee, a procedure with its own associated morbidities. Allograft tissue carries the risk of disease transmission and delayed biologic incorporation and also presents issues related to cost and availability. It also removes the native ACL tissue and the sensory nerve fibers (and thus neuromuscular function) of the ligament. Lastly, it replaces a complex, fan-shaped bundle of 17 different ligament fascicles with a single or double bundle of tendon fibers. The point-to-point graft is unable to restore the normal rotational kinematics of the knee. Some of these deficiencies may contribute to the premature degeneration of the joint, which occurs after ACL injury, even with ACL reconstruction.[2] Perhaps the most concerning problem, however, is the fact that even with ACL reconstruction, patients have a high risk for premature post-injury osteoarthritis. Even with the gold standard of treatment for ACL injury, as many as 78% of patients will have radiographic signs of arthritis 14 years after surgery.[2]

DEFINING THE ACL RESPONSE TO INJURY
Response in the Human ACL

The histologic response to injury in the human ACL has been found to be significantly different from that previously reported in the MCL. One study examined human ACL tissue before and after rupture[17,18] and compared the cellular responses in the ACL with those previously reported for the MCL.[6,19] Using histology and immunohistochemistry techniques, it was found that like MCL cells, the ACL cells within the ligament proliferate and the ligament revascularizes after rupture (**Fig. 2**).[6,18,19] Collagen production was also noted to continue within the ligament up to 1 year out from injury.[20] Cells in both the intact and ruptured ACL were found to migrate easily into a simulated wound site.[21–23]

However, the provisional scaffold that reconnected the torn collagen fascicles in the wound site of the MCL was missing in the ACL, where the 2 ends of the ruptured

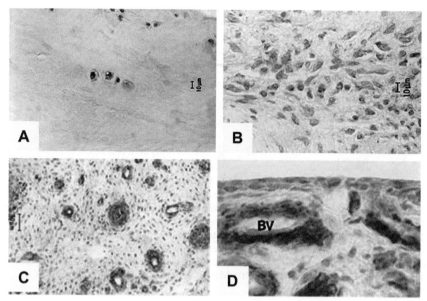

Fig. 2. Histologic response of the human ACL to rupture. (*A*) Histologic appearance of the normal ACL showing fibroblasts (blue nuclei; 40×). (*B*) Histologic appearance of ACL tissue 3 mo after rupture showing increased cell density in the ligament ends (40×). (*C*) Area of increased vessel density in ruptured ACL fragments at 3 mo after injury (20×). (*D*) Synovial layer that has reformed over the ligament ends at 8 wk after rupture (BV = blood vessel, 40×). Sections are immunohistochemistry for alpha-smooth muscle actin (SMA) where red demonstrates a positive stain for SMA, with a blue counter-stain for cell nuclei.[18]

ligament were simply churning around in synovial fluid and never able to reconnect.[18] Thus, it appeared that while the cells and vascularity of the ACL were capable of mounting a histologic healing response, there was no structural evidence of a filling in at the wound site in the ACL (**Fig. 3**).

Response in Animal Studies Comparing ACL and MCL

The observation that there was essentially no provisional scaffold formation or wound site filling between the ends of the ruptured human ACL led to additional in vivo studies comparing the ACL and MCL histologic response to injury in a mechanically stable and contained defect.[24] Central defects were created in extra-articular ligaments (MCL and/or patellar ligament) and an intra-articular ligament (ACL) in canine knees and the histologic response to injury evaluated at 3 days (n = 3), 7 days (n = 4), 21 days (n = 5), and 42 days (n = 5).

The findings in these studies were that MCL and patellar ligament defects exhibited far greater filling of the wound site and increased presence in the wound site of fibrinogen, fibronectin, platelet-derived growth factor-A (PDGF-A), transforming growth factor-beta1 (TGF-b1), fibroblast growth factor (FGF) and vonWillebrand's factor (vWF) when compared with ACL defects at all time points (**Fig. 4**).[25] Thus, this study supported the hypothesis that there is a lack of provisional scaffold found in the intra-articular wound site of the ACL, and this loss is also associated with a decreased presence of important extracellular matrix proteins and cytokines within the wound site of the ACL.

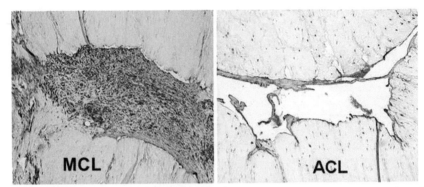

Fig. 3. Representative micrographs of slit wounds made with a modified Beaver blade in the center of the MCL and ACL 7 d earlier in a canine knee. Note that the MCL wound is filled with a provisional scaffolding material containing high amounts of multiple growth factors important in tissue healing (here, immunohistochemistry for FGF-2, where red is a positive stain). In the ACL wound, however, the defect remains unfilled, even after 7 d. (*Adapted from* Steiner ME, Murray MM, Rodeo SA. Strategies to improve anterior cruciate ligament healing and graft placement. Am J Sports Med 2008;36(1):176–89; with permission.)

NOVEL HYPOTHESIS FOR ETIOLOGY OF ACL NON-UNION

These findings in humans[17,18,20–22] and in the experimental large animal model[24–26] led to a unique hypothesis, namely, that perhaps it was this lack of provisional scaffold between the 2 ends of the torn ACL that was a key mechanism behind the failure of the ACL to heal. In the MCL and other comparable tissues that heal successfully outside of joints, the very first phase of the healing response is filling of the defect with a fibrin-platelet plug that bridges the wound edges.[19] This plug, or scaffold, is then subsequently invaded by reparative cells that remodel the scaffold into a healing

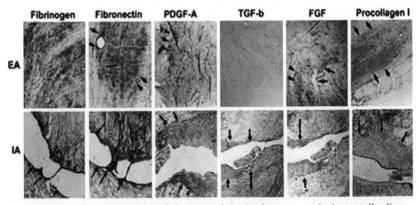

Fig. 4. Representative micrographs of the wound site in the extra-articular patellar ligament (EA row) and the intra-articular ACL (IA row) after 3 wk in vivo. Note the filling of the wound site in the EA ligament with an active repair process occurring within the provisional scaffold (*top row*). In contrast, the ACL wounds remain unfilled (*bottom row*). (*From* Murray MM, Spindler KP, Ballard P, et al. Enhanced histologic repair in a central wound in the anterior cruciate ligament with a collagen-platelet-rich plasma scaffold. J Orthop Res 2007;25(8):1007–17; with permission.)

fibrovascular scar (see **Fig. 3**). The formation of the early provisional scaffold is the first critical step in the wound healing process.

However, inside the joint, even though bleeding occurs after ACL injury, no fibrin-platelet plug is observed to form, even at the injury site (see **Fig. 3**).[27] One possible explanation for this finding is that circulating intra-articular plasmin breaks down the fibrin plug as fast as it can form. Recent work has shown that after trauma to the joint, the production of plasmin is upregulated through the increased secretion of urokinase plasminogen activator (**Fig. 5**).[28] With the additional circulating plasmin, the fibrin network is quickly destabilized within the joint environment and no fibrin-platelet plug forms.

This premature loss of the fibrin-platelet plug would have the significant clinical benefit of preventing overall joint scarring and stiffness (arthrofibrosis) and, thus, maintenance of joint mobility after injury. However, the degradation of the fibrin-platelet plug in the overall joint would also remove it prematurely from any wound sites. As the formation of the fibrin-platelet plug is the essential first step for wound healing of musculoskeletal tissue outside the joint[19], it is believed that the loss of this fibrin-platelet plug inside the joint is the key mechanism behind the failure of tissues in the joint (intra-articular tissues) to heal (**Fig. 6**). The hypothesis that the premature failure of the provisional scaffold is the impediment to ACL healing is an important change from previous mechanisms proposed for ACL non-union, which focused predominantly on the intrinsic cell and vascular responses.[11–13,15,29–34] Past research based on the cell-deficiency hypothesis has focused predominantly on stimulation of cells in vitro with growth factors or on cell transplantation into wound sites (including the use of stem cells and genetically modified cells). However, if it were failure of the provisional scaffold, an additional line of inquiry into the placement of a substitute scaffold itself would be a logical step (**Fig. 7**).

IN VITRO DEVELOPMENT OF A SUBSTITUTE SCAFFOLD

Based on early studies on the provisional scaffold failure in the ACL wound site in humans and animals, materials that might be useful in the ACL wound site were evaluated. The substitute scaffold would need to withstand the physical and mechanical

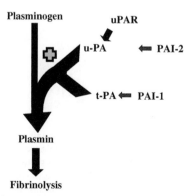

Fig. 5. Proposed pathway for accelerated fibrinolysis after joint injury. The increased secretion of urokinase plasminogen activator (u-PA) results in high levels of plasmin in the inflammatory synovial fluid. This is a likely mechanism for the accelerated fibrinolysis noted in the joint after injury. (PAI-1 and 2: Plasminogen activator inhibitor 1 and 2; t-PA: tissue plasminogen activator; uPAR: urokinase-type plasminogen activator receptor.)

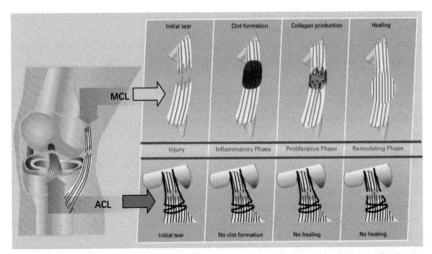

Fig. 6. Novel hypothesis of the failure of ACL healing. For the MCL which is outside the joint, injury is followed by formation of a provisional scaffold in the form of a fibrin clot. The scaffold is gradually remodeled as the tissue heals (*top row*). No fibrin clot is found at the injury site of the ACL, which is inside the knee joint. Without a provisional scaffold, the wound site remains empty and healing cannot proceed.

conditions of the intra-articular environment. The mechanical boundary conditions require that the scaffold be able to withstand the relatively high physiologic strains seen by the connective tissues of interest, strains which typically approach 3% during normal knee motion.[35] Enzymatically, the bridge would need to be resistant to degradation by circulating intra-articular inflammatory metabolites and proteolytic enzymes that are present after injury or surgery, including plasmin,[28] matrix metalloproteinases,[36] and glycosidases.[37] It is also likely that biologic stimuli would be required to successfully replicate the successful wound healing environment, either in the form of a single cytokine[38,39] (sufficiently upstream in the wound healing cascade) or in a group of growth factors, including the cohort released by platelets in other wound sites.

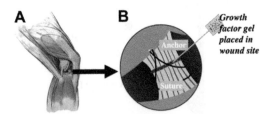

Fig. 7. (A) and (B). Schematic of the enhanced suture repair technique. (A) The location of the ACL between femur and tibia is illustrated. The enlarged view on the right (B) shows a transected ACL treated with suture repair, where the sutures are attached to an anchor in the bone at the femoral insertion site and then are passed through the longer distal ACL segment and tied to reapproximate the proximal and distal ACL segments. The growth factor hydrogel is introduced into the wound site to stimulate biologic repair. (A) View of the ACL position within the knee. (B) Schematic of suture repair supplemented with a growth factor gel. (*Reproduced from* Murray MM, Spindler KP, Abreu E, et al. Collagen-platelet rich plasma hydrogel enhances primary repair of the porcine anterior cruciate ligament. J Orthop Res 2007;25:81–91; with permission).

BIOLOGIC AUGMENTATION OF PRIMARY ACL REPAIR
Supplementation with Growth Factors

In vitro studies have demonstrated improved cellular proliferation and migration as well as increased collagen production rates with the addition of growth factors including platelet-derived growth factor (PDGF),[16,40] TGF-b,[40] and FGF.[29,40] In follow-up studies of these in vitro results, healing of the ACL using growth factors in animal models has also been studied.[39,41] Kobayashi and colleagues[41] noted improved filling and vascularity surrounding a central defect in a canine ACL model with implantation of a bFGF pellet; however, no biomechanical testing was performed in that study. In a study of MCL transection in a rabbit model, Spindler and colleagues[39] reported that the addition of TGF-b2 to the wound site resulted in an increase in scar size, but not scar strength.

Supplementing Structure Using Scaffolds

Healing of intra-articular defects using substitute provisional scaffolds is a recent area of interest. Defects in the ACL have been treated with synthetic scaffolds loaded with growth factors, including TGF-b,[41] and also with hyaluronic acid.[42] These techniques have had limited success, but unfortunately continue to have problems with implant-host integration, cell survival after transplantation, and degradation with time. Better results have been obtained with the use of collagen scaffolds loaded with platelets.

Hyaluronic Acid as a Scaffold Treatment

In a central defect rabbit model, Wiig and colleagues[42] reported improved covering of a central defect in the ACL with intra-articular injection of hyaluronic acid in a rabbit model. In that study, a greater angiogenic response was seen in the group of HA-treated ligaments. More type III collagen was produced in the ligaments treated with HA than in the group of ligaments treated with saline. No biomechanical testing was reported for that study.

Collagen–Platelet Composites

Recent studies have detailed the outcomes of treating a complete ACL transection with a suture repair augmented with a substitute scaffold. The complete transection model in the pig results in instability of the knee joint and provides a harsher healing environment that closely mimics the condition of the human knee after ACL rupture. In this study, bilateral ACL transections were performed in seven 30-kg Yorkshire pigs and repaired with a 4-stranded, absorbable suture repair (see **Fig. 7**).[43] In 5 animals, 1 of the repairs was augmented with placement of a collagen–platelet composite at the ACL transection site, whereas the contralateral knee had suture repair alone. No postoperative immobilization was used. After a 4-week healing period the animals underwent in vivo magnetic resonance imaging followed by euthanasia and immediate biomechanical testing. Six control knees with intact ACLs from 3 additional animals were used as an intact ACL control group. Supplementation of suture repair with a collagen–platelet composite resulted in the formation of a large scar mass in the region of the ACL. Load at yield, maximum load, and ACL tangent modulus were all significantly higher in the suture repairs augmented with collagen–platelet composite than in repairs performed with suture alone. This article concluded that biomechanical healing of the porcine ACL after complete transection and immediate suture repair can be enhanced at an early time point with use of a collagen–platelet composite placed in the wound site at the time of primary repair.[43]

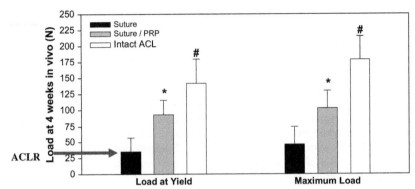

Fig. 8. Load at yield and maximum load for the 3 groups: suture repair alone (Suture), suture repair plus collagen–platelet composite (Suture/PRP), and intact ACLs (Intact ACL). Differences were observed between intact ACLs and each of the other 2 groups (denoted by #). Load at yield and maximum load were both significantly higher for suture repair plus collagen–platelet composite compared with suture repair alone as denoted by asterisks. Error bars represent standard deviations. Arrow designates yield strength of ACL reconstruction at a similar time point.[44] (*Adapted from* Steiner ME, Murray MM, Rodeo SA. Strategies to improve anterior cruciate ligament healing and graft placement. Am J Sports Med 2008;36(1):76–89; with permission.)

The results of this study demonstrated that primary repair using the collagen–platelet composite resulted in healing ligament strength that was over 50% of the intact ligament strength 4 weeks after repair. This strength compares favorably with the current gold standard of ACL reconstruction, where strengths at 3 to 4 weeks are under 25% of the intact ligament strength (**Fig. 8**).[44]

FUTURE DIRECTIONS

This first demonstration of histologic and biomechanical healing of the ACL will likely lead to entirely new fields of inquiry surrounding treatment of this important structure. Hypotheses regarding the influence of patient age or gender on repair outcome become interesting and important, as do questions regarding the ability to maintain "mechanical homeostasis" by stimulating sufficient anabolic cellular responses to generate wound strength, while at the same time, encouraging gradual catabolism of the provisional scaffold. It is also likely that the concentration of cellular components of the platelet-rich plasma (specifically platelets and leukocytes) significantly effect the cellular proliferation and migration into the wound site, as might the concentration of the extracellular matrix molecules within the substitute scaffold. One might hypothesize that changes in these fundamental cellular behaviors may result in significant changes in the mechanical, and functional, properties of this ligament. These are just a few of the questions that will likely be investigated over the next few years.

SUMMARY

The last decade of research into the potential of primary ACL repair has resulted in the discovery of a novel mechanism to explain the failure of the ACL to heal and the validation of several large animal models to test new techniques of repair in vivo. Further optimization of these techniques into a successful surgical procedure has the potential to alter the clinical treatment of ACL injuries.

ACKNOWLEDGMENTS

Funding was received from NIH grants AR052772, AR054099, and AR049346.

REFERENCES

1. Myer GD, Ford KR, Hewett T. Rationale and clinical techniques for anterior cruciate ligament injury prevention among female athletes. J Athl Train 2004;39:352–64. Available at: http://www.ncbi.nlm.nih.gov/entrez/query.fcgi?cmd=Retrieve&db=PubMed&dopt=Citation&list_uids=15592608.
2. Von Porat A, Roos EM, Roos H. High prevalence of osteoarthritis 14 years after an anterior cruciate ligament tear in male soccer players: a study of radiographic and patient relevant outcomes. Br J Sports Med 2004;38:263. Available at: http://www.ncbi.nlm.nih.gov/entrez/query.fcgi?cmd=Retrieve&db=PubMed&dopt=Citation&list_uids=15155422.
3. Sherman MF, Bonamo JR. Primary repair of the anterior cruciate ligament. Clin Sports Med 1988;7:739–50.
4. Kaplan N, Wickiewicz TL, Warren RF. Primary surgical treatment of anterior cruciate ligament ruptures: a long-term follow-up study. Am J Sports Med 1990;18: 254–358.
5. Feagin JA Jr, Curl WW. Isolated tear of the anterior cruciate ligament: 5-year follow-up study. Am J Sports Med 1976;4:95–100.
6. Woo SL, Vogrin TM, Abramowitch SD. Healing and repair of ligament injuries in the knee. J Am Acad Orthop Surg 2000;8:364–72.
7. Andrish J, Holmes R. Effects of synovial fluid on fibroblasts in tissue culture. Clin Orthop 1979;138:279–83.
8. Amiel D, Ishizue KK, Harwood FL, et al. Injury of the anterior cruciate ligament: the role of collagenase in ligament degeneration. J Orthop Res 1989;7:486–93. Available at: http://www.ncbi.nlm.nih.gov/entrez/query.fcgi?cmd=Retrieve&db=PubMed&dopt=Citation&list_uids=2544709.
9. Saris DB, Dhert WJ, Verbout AJ. Joint homeostasis. The discrepancy between old and fresh defects in cartilage repair. J Bone Joint Surg Br 2003;85:1067–76. Available at: http://www.ncbi.nlm.nih.gov/entrez/query.fcgi?cmd=Retrieve&db=PubMed&dopt=Citation&list_uids=14516049.
10. Wiig M, Amiel D, Ivarsson M, et al. Type I procollagen gene expression in normal and early healing of the medial collateral and anterior cruciate ligaments in rabbits: an in situ hybridization study. J Orthop Res 1991;9:374–82.
11. Lyon RM, Akeson WH, Amiel D, et al. Ultrastructural differences between the cells of the medical collateral and the anterior cruciate ligaments. Clin Orthop 1991;279–86. Available at: http://www.ncbi.nlm.nih.gov/entrez/query.fcgi?cmd=Retrieve&db=PubMed&dopt=Citation&list_uids=1934745.
12. Nagineni CN, Amiel D, Green MH, et al. Characterization of the intrinsic properties of the anterior cruciate and medial collateral ligament cells: an in vitro cell culture study. J Orthop Res 1992;10:465–75. Available at: http://www.ncbi.nlm.nih.gov/entrez/query.fcgi?cmd=Retrieve&db=PubMed&dopt=Citation&list_uids=1613622.
13. Gesink DS, Pacheco HO, Kuiper SD, et al. Immunohistochemical localization of beta 1-integrins in anterior cruciate and medial collateral ligaments of human and rabbit. J Orthop Res 1992;10:596–9. Available at: http://www.ncbi.nlm.nih.gov/entrez/query.fcgi?cmd=Retrieve&db=PubMed&dopt=Citation&list_uids=1377240.
14. Schreck PJ, Kitabayashi LR, Amiel D, et al. Integrin display increases in the wounded rabbit medial collateral ligament but not the wounded anterior cruciate ligament.

J Orthop Res 1995;13:174–83. Available at: http://www.ncbi.nlm.nih.gov/entrez/query.fcgi?cmd=Retrieve&db=PubMed&dopt=Citation&list_uids=7722754.

15. Lee J, Harwood FL, Akeson WH, et al. Growth factor expression in healing rabbit medial collateral and anterior cruciate ligaments. Iowa Orthop J 1998;18:19–25. Available at: http://www.ncbi.nlm.nih.gov/entrez/query.fcgi?cmd=Retrieve&db=PubMed&dopt=Citation&list_uids=9807704.

16. Kobayashi K, Healey RM, Sah RL, et al. Novel method for the quantitative assessment of cell migration: a study on the motility of rabbit anterior cruciate (ACL) and medial collateral ligament (MCL) cells. Tissue Eng 2000;6:29–38. Available at: http://www.ncbi.nlm.nih.gov/entrez/query.fcgi?cmd=Retrieve&db=PubMed&dopt=Citation&list_uids=10941198.

17. Murray MM, Spector M. Fibroblast distribution in the anteromedial bundle of the human anterior cruciate ligament: the presence of alpha-smooth muscle actin-positive cells. J Orthop Res 1999;17:18–27.

18. Murray MM, Martin SD, Martin TL, et al. Histological changes in the human anterior cruciate ligament after rupture. J Bone Joint Surg Am 2000;82-A:1387–97.

19. Frank C, Amiel D, Akeson WH. Healing of the medial collateral ligament of the knee. A morphological and biochemical assessment in rabbits. Acta Orthop Scand 1983;54:917–23.

20. Spindler KP, Clark SW, Nanney LB, et al. Expression of collagen and matrix metalloproteinases in ruptured human anterior cruciate ligament: an in situ hybridization study. J Orthop Res 1996;14:857–61.

21. Murray MM, Martin SD, Spector M. Migration of cells from human anterior cruciate ligament explants into collagen-glycosaminoglycan scaffolds. J Orthop Res 2000;18:557–64.

22. Murray MM, Spector M. The migration of cells from the ruptured human anterior cruciate ligament into collagen-glycosaminoglycan regeneration templates in vitro. Biomaterials 2001;22:2393–402.

23. Steiner ME, Murray MM, Rodeo SA. Strategies to improve anterior cruciate ligament healing and graft placement. Am J Sports Med 2008;36:176–89. Available at: http://www.ncbi.nlm.nih.gov/entrez/query.fcgi?cmd=Retrieve&db=PubMed&dopt=Citation&list_uids=18166680.

24. Spindler KP, Murray MM, Devin C, et al. The central ACL defect as a model for failure of intra-articular healing. J Orthop Res 2006;24:401–6. Available at: http://www.ncbi.nlm.nih.gov/entrez/query.fcgi?cmd=Retrieve&db=PubMed&dopt=Citation&list_uids=16479574.

25. Murray MM, Spindler KP, Ballard P, et al. Enhanced histologic repair in a central wound in the anterior cruciate ligament with a collagen-platelet-rich plasma scaffold. J Orthop Res; 2007. Available at: http://www.ncbi.nlm.nih.gov/entrez/query.fcgi?cmd=Retrieve&db=PubMed&dopt=Citation&list_uids=17415785.

26. Murray MM, Spindler KP, Devin C, et al. Use of a collagen-platelet rich plasma scaffold to stimulate healing of a central defect in the canine ACL. J Orthop Res 2006;24:820–30. Available at: http://www.ncbi.nlm.nih.gov/entrez/query.fcgi?cmd=Retrieve&db=PubMed&dopt=Citation&list_uids=16555312.

27. Harrold AJ. The defect of blood coagulation in joints. J Clin Pathol 1961;14:305–8.

28. Rosc D, Powierza W, Zastawna E, et al. Post-traumatic plasminogenesis in intra-articular exudate in the knee joint. Med Sci Monit 2002;8:CR371–8.

29. Amiel D, Nagineni CN, Choi SH, et al. Intrinsic properties of ACL and MCL cells and their responses to growth factors. Med Sci Sports Exerc 1995;27:844–51.

30. Chen H, Tang Y, Li S, et al. Biologic characteristics of fibroblast cells cultured from the knee ligaments. Chin J Traumatol 2002;5:92–6.

31. Geiger MH, Amiel D, Green MH, et al. Rates of migration of ACL and MCL derived fibroblasts. Orthop Trans 1992;17:75.
32. Geiger MH, Green MH, Monosov A, et al. An in vitro assay of anterior cruciate ligament (ACL) and medial collateral ligament (MCL) cell migration. Connect Tissue Res 1994;30:215–24.
33. Spindler KP, Imro AK, Mayes CE, et al. Patellar tendon and anterior cruciate ligament have different mitogenic responses to platelet-derived growth factor and transforming growth factor beta. J Orthop Res 1996;14:542–6.
34. Spindler KP, Andrish JT, Miller RR, et al. Distribution of cellular repopulation and collagen synthesis in a canine anterior cruciate ligament autograft. J Orthop Res 1996;14:384–9.
35. Heijne A, Fleming BC, Renstrom PA, et al. Strain on the anterior cruciate ligament during closed kinetic chain exercises. Med Sci Sports Exerc 2004;36:935–41. Available at: http://www.ncbi.nlm.nih.gov/entrez/query.fcgi?cmd=Retrieve&db=PubMed&dopt=Citation&list_uids=15179161.
36. Fernandes JC, Martel-Pelletier J, Pelletier JP. The role of cytokines in osteoarthritis pathophysiology. Biorheology 2002;39:237–46. Available at: http://www.ncbi.nlm.nih.gov/entrez/query.fcgi?cmd=Retrieve&db=PubMed&dopt=Citation&list_uids=12082286.
37. Shikhman AR, Brinson DC, Lotz M. Profile of glycosaminoglycan-degrading glycosidases and glycoside sulfatases secreted by human articular chondrocytes in homeostasis and inflammation. Arthritis Rheum 2000;43:1307–14. Available at: http://www.ncbi.nlm.nih.gov/entrez/query.fcgi?cmd=Retrieve&db=PubMed&dopt=Citation&list_uids=10857789.
38. Spindler KP, Dawson JM, Stahlman GC, et al. Collagen expression and biomechanical response to human recombinant transforming growth factor beta (rhTGF-beta2) in the healing rabbit MCL. J Orthop Res 2002;20:318–24.
39. Spindler KP, Murray MM, Detwiler KB, et al. The biomechanical response to doses of TGF-beta 2 in the healing rabbit medial collateral ligament. J Orthop Res 2003;21:245–9.
40. Meaney Murray M, Rice K, Wright RJ, et al. The effect of selected growth factors on human anterior cruciate ligament cell interactions with a three-dimensional collagen-GAG scaffold. J Orthop Res 2003;21:238–44.
41. Kobayashi D, Kurosaka M, Yoshiya S, et al. Effect of basic fibroblast growth factor on the healing of defects in the canine anterior cruciate ligament. Knee Surg Sports Traumatol Arthrosc 1997;5:189–94. Available at: http://www.ncbi.nlm.nih.gov/entrez/query.fcgi?cmd=Retrieve&db=PubMed&dopt=Citation&list_uids=9335032.
42. Wiig ME, Amiel D, VandeBerg J, et al. The early effect of high molecular weight hyaluronan (hyaluronic acid) on anterior cruciate ligament healing: an experimental study in rabbits. J Orthop Res 1990;8:425–34. Available at: http://www.ncbi.nlm.nih.gov/entrez/query.fcgi?cmd=Retrieve&db=PubMed&dopt=Citation&list_uids=2324860.
43. Murray MM, Spindler KP, Abreu E, et al. Collagen-platelet rich plasma hydrogel enhances primary repair of the porcine anterior cruciate ligament. J Orthop Res 2007;25:81–91. Available at: http://www.ncbi.nlm.nih.gov/entrez/query.fcgi?cmd=Retrieve&db=PubMed&dopt=Citation&list_uids=17031861.
44. Hunt P, Scheffler SU, Unterhauser FN, et al. A model of soft-tissue graft anterior cruciate ligament reconstruction in sheep. Arch Orthop Trauma Surg 2005;125:238–48. Available at: http://www.ncbi.nlm.nih.gov/entrez/query.fcgi?cmd=Retrieve&db=PubMed&dopt=Citation&list_uids=15024579.

Advances in Rehabilitation and Performance Testing

William Cates, PT, DPT, ES*, John Cavanaugh, PT, Med, ATC

KEYWORDS

• Functional • Performance • Tests • Rehabilitation • Sports

Specialized testing procedures allow rehabilitation clinicians and strength and conditioning specialists to measure progress and functional level. Testing will ensure a safe progression throughout the rehabilitative course by providing the needed criteria for advancement. Performance testing quantifies the pure physical nature of athletic performance. Successful rehabilitation can be attained only by following a functional progression. Testing procedures also follow a progression, which begins with basic measures and progresses to functional tests of increasing difficulty that include sports-specific testing before returning to field play. Clinical tests provide both quantitative and qualitative information. These tests not only quantify physiologic response to rehabilitation but also allow the clinician to provide qualitative feedback to an individual during a specific activity. Balance, strength, power, cardiovascular endurance, functional movement, as well as the component of apprehension with sport-specific activity are important and valuable measures in prevention, rehabilitation, and performance programs.

Rehabilitation clinicians and strength and conditioning specialists are vital to an athlete during rehabilitation after an injury or when training to enhance his or her competitive performance. Rehabilitation clinicians serve to prepare an athlete for return to sport after injury. Strength and conditioning specialists serve to improve an athlete's physical performance by providing a sports-specific individualized fitness program. The use of specialized testing procedures allows these professionals to measure progress and functional level.

Rehabilitation testing will ensure a safe progression throughout the rehabilitative course by providing the necessary criteria for advancement. Performance testing quantifies the pure physical nature of athletic performance. Performance in any sport is determined by the athlete's technical, tactical, physiologic, and psychosocial characteristics.[1] Rehabilitation clinicians and strength and conditioning specialists should

The Hospital for Special Surgery, Sports Rehabilitation and Performance Center, 535 E 70th Street, New York, NY 10021, USA
* Corresponding author.
E-mail address: catesw@hss.edu (W. Cates).

Clin Sports Med 28 (2009) 63–76
doi:10.1016/j.csm.2008.09.003
0278-5919/08/$ – see front matter © 2008 Elsevier Inc. All rights reserved.
sportsmed.theclinics.com

be familiar with current practices and standardizations of tests and measures to provide an accurate prediction model for the successful return of an athlete to his or her sport. These tests and measures encompass a vast array of skill sets and body systems. This article discusses the most recent advances in rehabilitation and performance testing, which use updated approaches and thought processes in their design.

Successful rehabilitation can be attained only by following a functional progression. Kegerreis[2] has defined a functional progression as "an ordered sequence of activities enabling the acquisition or reacquisition of skills required for the safe, effective performance of athletic endeavors." To ensure adherence to this concept, graded testing procedures should be employed. Davies describes a functional testing algorithm (FTA) (**Table 1**) that begins with basic measures and progresses to functional tests of increasing difficulty, which include sports-specific testing before returning to field play.[3] The progression model is designed to increase the stresses placed on the athlete by providing different functional testing maneuvers, which require an increase in motor control. These tests can be performed in the clinic beginning with basic functional movements.

On successful completion of the clinical tests and clearance from the referring physician, the athlete may progress to a pre-participation examination that consists of sports-specific field tests. These tests incorporate sport specific movements and are aligned with the skill set needed for participation in a particular sport. The athlete's sport and his/her specialty within that sport will determine the testing procedures that are used.

Within the FTA progression model, clinical tests address both qualitative and quantitative data. Qualitative data are defined as the attributes of movement during a particular task, whereas quantitative data are defined as numerical results obtained from a given test measurement. In recent years, clinicians have accepted the importance of functional training. Many clinicians have modified the rehabilitation model to focus on more than just pure isolated movement exercises.[4] The improvement in the quality of movement will increase the efficiency of the athletic movement and thus carry over onto the playing field. Therefore, a new approach to performance testing that includes the standardization of qualitative data should be used.

Obtaining quantitative data is inherent and necessary in athletic endeavors. The standardized data that quantitative tests produce are applicable at tryouts or combines when comparing the performance of athletes. They also provide a way to make comparisons between norms to determine an athlete's level of fitness or categorize athletic potential. In the clinical setting, standardized tests help to diagnose specific areas of weakness that may not be detectable with remedial testing

Table 1 Functional testing algorithm	
Yo-Yo tests Hop tests	Field Tests
Isoinertial testing Isokinetic testing Step-down test	Strength/Power
Balance testing Basic measurements	Basic Tests

Data from Davies G, Wilk K, Ellenbecker T. Assessment of strength. In: Malone TR, McPoil TG, Nitz AJ, editors. Orthopedic and sports physical therapy. 3rd edition. St. Louis (MO): Mosby; 1997. p. 231.

procedures. For example, the sensitivity of isokinetic dynamometry allows identification of changes in muscular power and strength between limbs, which may have been otherwise undetectable by basic manual muscle testing techniques.[3] These data can then be used to guide recommendations for return to sport or determine the next progressions in a rehabilitation program.

CLINICAL TESTS FOR REHABILITATION PROGRESSION

As previously discussed, clinical tests provide information regarding the level of progression the athlete has obtained within the rehabilitative process. Clinical tests also provide feedback to an athlete by identifying specific physical impairments. These tests must not only quantify physiologic response to rehabilitation but also allow the clinician to provide qualitative feedback to an individual during a specific activity.

BALANCE

Balance has been defined as the process of maintaining the center of gravity (COG) within the body's base of support.[5] The ability to maintain postural control involves multiple neurologic pathways. Afferent information received from the body's vestibular, visual, and somatosensory systems determine the corrective postural strategies employed to maintain balance. Proprioception is a precursor of good balance and adequate function.[6] Proprioception has been defined as a specialized variation of the sensory modality of touch, which includes the sensation of joint movement (kinesthesia) and joint position (joint position sense).[7] If proprioception is altered, a direct effect on balance can be expected.

Postural stability and kinesthetic awareness are important during athletic activities, such as running and cutting.[8] These abilities may be adversely affected by musculoskeletal injury, delaying the rehabilitation progress and impeding sports performance.

Clinical assessment of static and dynamic balance may be performed using computerized instrumentation on the NeuroCom Balance Master System (**Fig. 1**) and the Biodex Balance System (**Fig. 2**), respectively. These machines provide a high degree of statistical validity and reliability in determining postural sway differences between limbs.[9,10] They have been proven to have test-retest reliability of lower extremity functional instability measures involving testing situations of varying complexity.[11]

These machines are not readily available in all treatment settings, so other reliable methods of testing have been used. Star excursion balance test (SEBT) has been shown to be reliable and valid in determining postural deficits and is used to evaluate dynamic balance.[8,12] During this test, the patient is required to stand on 1 leg while reaching in different directions with the other leg along diagonal lines marked on the ground. The distance that is attained in each direction is recorded and interpreted as representation of dynamic balance.

In an attempt to identify athletes with a greater risk for lower extremity injury, Plisky and colleagues[12] examined the relationship between SEBT reach distance and lower extremity injury among high school basketball players. Results of the study revealed that a decreased normalized right composite reach distance and greater anterior right/left reach distance difference on the SEBT predicted lower extremity injury. This concept has several implications in terms of likelihood of injury for either limb. The first possibility is that the proficient limb might alter how the athlete reacts to competitive situations, causing increased stress to the more proficient limb. The second possibility is that the more adept extremity may absorb excessive force due to instability resulting from poor balance on the less adept extremity. The final possibility is

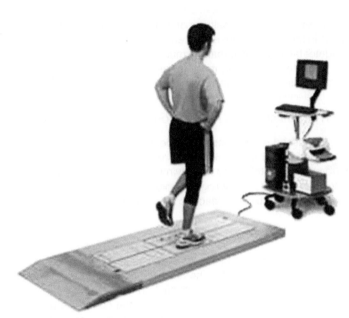

Fig.1. Static balance testing using the NeuroCom balance master system (NeuroCom International Inc. Clackamas, OR).

that the less adept lower extremity may not provide a stable platform on which to pivot or land.

This information allows rehabilitation clinicians and strength and conditioning specialists to be aware of weaknesses in players and the opportunity to take preemptive measures to avoid player injury.

STRENGTH ASSESSMENT

The assessment of lower extremity strength is a vital guideline in the safe progression of a patient throughout a rehabilitation program. Step-down tests have proven to be reliable and valid measurements to assess lower extremity strength.[13–15]

FORWARD STEP-DOWN TEST

A modification of the Step Up-and-Over Test[9] described by Neurocom, is the Forward step-down test.[13] This test can be used earlier in the treatment paradigm to assess early single-leg function of the knee extensor muscle group.

The Forward Step-Down Test uses force plate technology to quantify the impact of descent during a forward step down from an 8-" step (**Fig. 3**) Measurements of the amount of vertical impact that occurs from the contact" of the contralateral limb are recorded. This measurement allows the clinician to determine the eccentric muscle strength of the limb that is performing the action of lowering the body to the ground. An increase in vertical impact scores demonstrates a loss of motor control coinciding with weakness in the knee extensor muscle group. A mean impact index of 10% body weight and a limb symmetry of 85% have been reported as normative values.[13]

Additionally, the clinician should closely observe the quality of movement that the subject demonstrates. Qualitative assessment of the movement, including

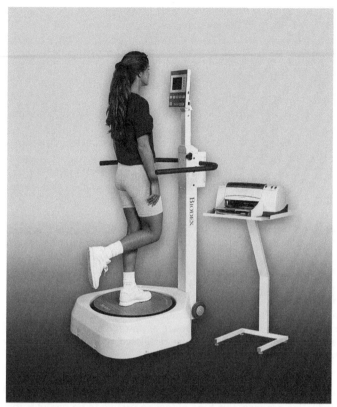

Fig. 2. Dynamic balance testing using the Biodex balance master system (Biodex Corporation, Shirley, NY).

contralateral hip drop, ipsilateral hip hike, increased valgus of the knee, and increased plantar flexion (reaching) of the contralateral foot all demonstrate faulty movement patterns. These compensatory qualitative responses should be used to provide feedback to the athlete. If these responses are detected, advancement into another stage of rehabilitation can be discouraged until selective criteria for completion of the test are met.

The single-leg step-down test has also been proven to be useful in the identification of injury susceptibility. Earl and colleagues[14] examined the differences in knee, hip, and ankle kinematics in patients using drop jump and single-leg step-down tests. The tests revealed that the drop jump produced greater knee abduction than the single-leg step down and is appropriate for evaluating anterior cruciate ligament (ACL) risk in athletes. The single-leg step down produced greater motion in the frontal and transverse planes at the ankle and hip and is appropriate for evaluating control of the hip. They concluded that both tests should be used together in the evaluation and examination of injury risk among athletes.

ISOKINETICS

Isokinetic dynamometry has been used since the 1960s to provide strength and power assessment of the elite athlete.[16] Isokinetics has also been instrumental in providing

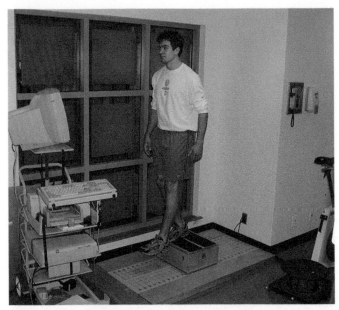

Fig. 3. Forward step-down test: The patient steps down an 8″ step onto the force plate (Balance Master System) as slowly and as controlled as possible on each leg. Three trials are recorded. Mean impact and limb symmetry are calculated and interpreted. Lower extremity control is observed for deviations.

an effective tool in the assessment of the injured athlete returning to sport.[3] Throughout the rehabilitative process, this type of testing proves to be useful in the functional progression model because of the quantitative, objective data it provides (**Fig. 4**). The objective data that are obtained provide a comprehensive assessment of muscle

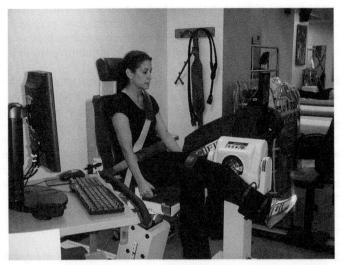

Fig. 4. Isokinetic knee testing on Biodex System 4 (Biodex Corporation, Shirley, NY).

torque, work, power, and acceleration. These measures, especially when comparing muscular strength of an injured extremity versus an uninjured extremity, provide pertinent information regarding the athlete's response to rehabilitation.[17] The nature of isokinetics provides a more controlled platform from which to test. This allows clinicians to test athletes with fewer degrees of freedom, allowing for a safer method to gain quantitative data on muscular strength and performance.

However, the validity of isokinetics in the assessment of athletic performance has been questioned in recent studies.[18–22] Correlating the information obtained from this type of testing to athletic performance may be less useful due to the nature of the test. Typical isokinetics use isolated open-chain movements, which may be deemed less functional, especially when performed in a single plane of movement. On the contrary, athletic activities consist of closed-chain movements that are multi-plane and multi-joint in nature.[23]

Therefore, isokinetics is a useful tool when assessing a patient progressing through a rehabilitation program. However, because the testing movement patterns involve joint isolation, the testing procedure is limited when attempting to assess the true sports performance of an athlete.

HOP TESTS

The hop test was developed by Daniel and colleagues[24] and was designed to gauge both strength and confidence in the involved leg. In contrast to isokinetic testing, the hop test is inexpensive to administer and uses movements of a more athletic-based nature. Various 1-legged tests for distance, 2-legged tests, and vertical jumps have also been established as measurements of the return to a functional level and the patient's perception of knee function.[25]

Measurement reliability has been reported for various hop-test procedures in non-impaired subjects, in impaired subjects who have undergone ACL reconstruction, and also in subjects with chronic ankle instability (CAI).[26–30] An important reason for the continued use of the hop test in rehabilitation is its proven statistical validity. Several studies have reported intraclass correlation coefficient (ICCs) of high levels. In non-impaired individuals, ICCs averaged to be 0.94 for the single-hop test and ranged from 0.88 to 0.97 in subjects who underwent ACL reconstruction.[26,28,29]

A combination of 4 different hop tests described by Noyes and colleagues[31] may be particularly suitable as a clinical-based outcome measure for patients who undergo rehabilitation after ACL reconstructive surgery. The tests involve a variety of movement principles (including speed, direction change, rebound, and acceleration-deceleration) that imitate the demands of dynamic knee stability during athletic sports activities and are recommended for the patient to return to such activity.[17,20,29,32,33] This series of hop tests involves a single hop for distance, a 6-m timed hop, a triple hop for distance, and crossover hops for distance (**Fig. 5**). Measurements are obtained from both the operative and nonoperative extremities so that test performance on the impaired limb can be expressed as a percentage of test performance on the non-impaired limb, termed the "limb symmetry index" or LSI.[32]

More recently, clinicians such as Augustsson and colleagues[33] and Gustavsson and colleagues[34] have stated that even the conditions under which patients perform hop tests can greatly influence the validity and outcome of performance. Augustsson and colleagues noted that although most sports injuries occur at the end of a sporting event, when the athlete is fatigued, patients are typically examined for return to sports using functional tests performed under non-fatigued conditions. They studied patients under both non-fatigued and fatigued conditions using a single-leg hop test for

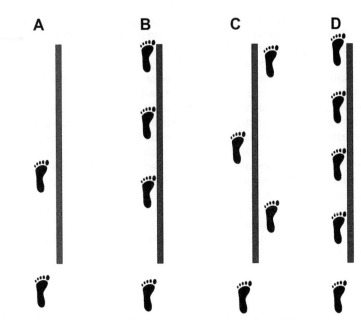

Fig. 5. Functional hop tests. A, Single-leg hop for distance; B, Triple hop for distance; C, Crossover triple hop for distance; D, One-legged timed hop.

distance. Their results showed that although no patients demonstrated abnormal hop test symmetry when non-fatigued 11 months post-operatively, two-thirds showed abnormal hop symmetry under fatigued test conditions. Furthermore, they found that patients are not fully rehabilitated 11 months after ACL construction. These findings have direct implications on clinicians' use of the hop test and potential recommendations of return to sport.

Elaborating on the findings of Augustsson, Gustavsson and colleagues conducted a study to prove that a test battery evaluating different hop qualities (ie, maximum single-hop performance, as well as hop performance while developing fatigue) increases the opportunity to detect inconsistencies in hop performance (ie, increase the test sensitivity) compared with using only a single-hop test. After testing 5 different single-leg hop tests, they found that 3 of the 5 tests had a high ability to discriminate between the hop performance of the injured and the uninjured side both in patients 6 months after ACL reconstruction and in patients 11 months after an ACL injury. The 3 hop tests chosen for their test battery are the vertical jump, the hop for distance, and the side hop. Using these 3 tests, it was observed that among patients who had undergone ACL reconstructive surgery, 54% of patients obtained an abnormal LSI in all 3 tests and 91% obtained abnormal LSI values in at least 1 of the 3 tests. It was also found that the test battery produced higher values, in terms of test-retest reliability, sensitivity, and accuracy, than those with any of the 3 hop tests individually.[34] This test battery may help in the process of deciding whether and when an athlete can return to strenuous physical activities after an ACL injury or reconstruction.

FUNCTIONAL MOVEMENT SCREEN

The concept of the FMS system was born from the realization that a significant number of athletes and individuals perform high-level activities with inefficient fundamental movements. Individuals compensate for poor movement patterns by training around their pre-existing movement impairment or by not training their weakness during strength or conditioning programs. FMS identifies abnormalities in fundamental movements and allows a clinician to address them. When completed, the athlete or individual will have a better understanding of his or her own inefficient movements, which in turn will lead to improved performance, and ultimately decrease injury potential.[4]

The FMS consists of 7 fundamental movement patterns that require a balance of mobility and stability. These movement patterns are designed to provide observable performance of basic locomotor, manipulative, and stabilizing movements. Placed in extreme positions, the tests reveal weaknesses and imbalances where stability and mobility are not appropriately used (**Fig. 6**). The 7 movement patterns are

- Deep squat
- Hurdle step
- In-line lunge
- Shoulder mobility
- Active straight leg raise
- Trunk stability push-up
- Rotary stability

The scoring of the FMS consists of 4 grades. Scores are simple in philosophy and range from 3, completion of the movement without any compensation to zero, wherein pain is present anywhere in the body during the movement. Five of the 7 movements test both the right and left sides, so it is important that both sides are scored. A difference in score between limbs indicates an imbalance and should be addressed with the conditioning plan or rehabilitation.[4]

The most important aspect of the FMS in terms of athletic performance is its ability to preemptively identify and thus address physical impairments in athletes, minimizing or eliminating injuries. In an attempt to examine injury risk factors in professional football players, Kiesel and colleagues[35] used the FMS to determine the relationship between the players' scores and the likelihood of serious injury. The study revealed that if

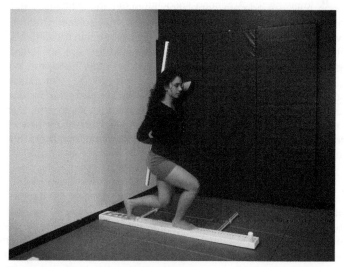

Fig. 6. Functional movement screen: in-line lunge.

a player had an FMS score of 14 or less, his or her probability of suffering a serious injury increased from 15% to 51%. The findings of this study suggest the possibility that the application of FMS scores paired with preventive rehabilitation can help minimize the likelihood of sports-related injuries for all athletes.

VERTICAL JUMP TEST

To more fully understand recent advancements in the vertical jump test, the concept of isoinertial strength must first be discussed. In contrast to isometric, isokinetic, and isotonic assessments, isoinertial is more closely reflected in the underlying muscular effort throughout a weight lifting-type task. In other words, isoinertial loading implies a constant resistance to motion rather than merely a constant resistance or load throughout the lift.[36,37] Murphy and colleagues[38] observed that movements in athletic settings involve the acceleration and deceleration of a constant mass about the associated joints or articulations. Given this fact, it has been suggested that the assessment of isoinertial strength should be an important tool for diagnosis and for the designing of appropriate strength-training programs for athletes.[38,39]

Advances in vertical jump testing have placed emphasis on digital technology and precision rather than on remedial vane/slat apparatus. More technologically advanced forms of the vertical jump test use force plates and timing mats, which provide precise and objective data in digital format.

In contrast to field hop tests (ie, the single-leg hop test for distance), the vertical jump force test (VJFT) addresses the measurement of force production. In a study conducted by Impellizzeri and colleagues,[40] a VJFT was used consisting of the measurement of vertical countermovement during jumping with both legs. The purposes of the study included the examination of the correlation between the VJFT and other measures of lower extremity strength, including isokinetic knee extension and isometric leg press. The isometric leg press was measured by attaching a force plate onto a horizontal leg press and recording a subject's single-leg maximal isometric contraction.[40]

The VJFT measurement was obtained by recording the vertical peak force produced by either the left or the right leg during a vertical jump. The results showed that there was only a moderate correlation between the VJFT and the isokinetic knee extension. This is explained by the fact that the isokinetic test isolates the knee joint, which is commonly observed with most open-chain movements. This suggests that the VJFT and the isokinetic knee-extension test are not interchangeable when assessing bilateral strength asymmetry. On the other hand, the isometric leg press test is more closed chain in nature and employs knee joint muscles as well as the muscles acting at the hip and ankle joints. This suggests that isokinetic testing should be used when assessing specific muscles around a single joint. Subsequently VJFT and other similarly designed closed-chain tests should be used to provide a comprehensive measure of strength to assess movements that more closely mimic functional activities of sport.

YO-YO TEST

Once an athlete or patient is able to participate in field tests after rehabilitation, the strength and conditioning specialist may want to test various aspects of performance. A simple form of tests are the 'yo-yo' tests, in which the physical capacity of the athlete is evaluated in a quick and efficient manner. The tests consist of running activities that are relevant to many sports.

Two markers are positioned on the ground 20 m apart and an audio CD is played. The participant runs like a yo-yo back and forth between the markers at specified speeds that are controlled by the CD. The speed is continuously and regularly increased, and when the individual can no longer maintain the speed, the test is terminated. The results of the test (**Fig. 7**) are determined by the distance covered during the test.[1]

Other forms of the yo-yo test exist to not exhaust the participant or for patients who are still in the rehabilitative stage of recovery. In these cases, a yo-yo test is administered that allows the participant to stop and rest after a given time period, and the change in heart rate is documented to evaluate cardiovascular condition.[1]

In total, there are 3 yo-yo tests. The yo-yo endurance test ranges in time from 5 to 15 minutes and is used to evaluate the ability of the participant to work continuously for an extended period of time. This test is applicable for individuals participating in endurance exercise such as distance running.[1] The other 2 tests, namely, the yo-yo intermittent endurance test and the yo-yo intermittent recovery test, have participants performing intermittent exercise and measure an individual's ability to repeatedly perform intense exercise.[1,41]

The yo-yo intermittent endurance test (Yo-Yo IR level 1) ranges from 10 to 20 minutes and is composed of approximately 5- to 18-second intervals of running interspersed with regular 5-second periods of rest.[1] This test evaluates a participant's ability to perform repeated intervals over a longer period of time, leading to a maximum level of activation of the aerobic system. This test is beneficial for the athlete who performs interval sports, such as tennis, soccer, and basketball.

The yo-yo intermittent recovery test level 2 (Yo-Yo IR 2) lasts 2 to 15 minutes and concentrates on the ability of the patient to recover after intense exercise with a substantial contribution from the anaerobic system.[41] Between each exercise period (ranging from 5–15 seconds) there is a 10-second pause. This test is well suited for athletes participating in sports that require periods of intense exertion following short recovery periods. Performing in sports in which the ability to perform intensive exercise after short recovery periods is essential to a positive outcome in competition. Such sports include football, soccer, and ice hockey.

The relationships between the results of yo-yo tests and athletic performance have been examined only in a few studies.[41–43] Krutstrup and colleagues[43] conducted a study of elite female athletes. The results indicated a significant correlation between high-intensity running at the end of each game half and the yo-yo intermittent test. This signifies that the test appears to be a useful tool in the evaluation of match-related physical capacity of soccer players.

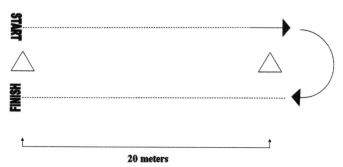

Fig. 7. Yo-yo intermittent test.

SUMMARY

Athletes continue to strive to maximize their physical and physiologic abilities to improve performance during competition. This dictates the need to assess their physical capacity to prepare them for return from an injury or to institute strength and conditioning programs. Rehabilitation clinicians and strength and conditioning specialists serve to provide specific assessments that identify qualitative and quantitative information pertinent for athletic performance enhancement. These assessments must demonstrate variability in movement patterns to effectively evaluate sports-specific functional movements during play. Improvements of these testing techniques are important due to the continually progressing nature of athletics. Increasing the number of valid tests during a clinical or performance evaluation will ultimately increase the specificity and utility of the results.

REFERENCES

1. McHugh M, Bangsbo J, Lexell J. Principles of rehabilitation following sports injury: sports-specific performance testing. In: Kjaes M, Krogsguard M, Magnusson P, et al, editors. Textbook of sports medicine. Oxford (United Kingdom): Blackwell Science; 2003. p. 201–25.
2. Kegerreis S. The construction and implementation of a functional progression as a component of athletic rehabilitation. J Orthop Sports Phys Ther 1983;14–9.
3. Davies G, Wilk K, Ellenbecker T. Assessment of strength. In: Malone TR, McPoil TG, Nitz AJ, editors. Orthopedic and sports physical therapy. 3rd edition. St. Louis (MO): Mosby; 1997. p. 225–57.
4. Cook G, Burton L, Hoogenboom B. Pre-participation screening: the use of fundamental movements as an assessment of function-part 1. North American Journal of Sports Physical Therapy 2006;1(2):62–72.
5. Nashner L. Sensory, neuromuscular and biomechanical contributions to human balance. In: Duncan PW, editor. Balance: proceedings of the APTA forum. Alexandria (VA): APTA; 1986.
6. Voight M, Blackburn T. Proprioception and balance training and testing following injury. In: Ellenbecker TS, editor. Knee ligament rehabilitation. Philadelphia: Churchill Livingston; 2000. p. 361–85.
7. Ergen E, Ulkar B. Proprioception and ankle injuries in soccer. Clin Sports Med 2008;27:195–217.
8. Kinzey S, Armstrong C. The reliability of the Star-excursion test in assessing dynamic balance. J Orthop Sports Phys Ther 1998;27(5):356–60.
9. Objective quantification of balance and mobility. Clackamas (OR): NeuroCom International, Inc; 2001.
10. Cachupe WC, Shifflett B, Kahanov L, et al. Reliability of Biodex balance system measures. Human performance department. San Jose State University; June 2000 [biodex 91–198].
11. Birmingham TB. Test-retest reliability of lower extremity functional instability measures. Clin J Sport Med 2000;10:264–8.
12. Plisky P, Rauh M, Kaminski TW, et al. Star Excursion Balance test as a predictor of lower extremity injury in high school basketball players. J Orthop Sports Phys Ther 2006;36(12):911–9.
13. Cavanaugh J, Stump T. Forward step down test. J Orthop Sports Phys Ther 2000; 30(1):A-46.

14. Earl J, Monteiro S, Snyder K. Differences in lower extremity kinematics between a bilateral drop-vertical jump and a single-leg step-down. J Orthop Sports Phys Ther 2007;37(5):245–52.
15. Chmielewski T, Hodges M, Horodyski M, et al. Investigation of clinician agreement in evaluating movement quality during unilateral lower extremity functional tasks: a comparison of 2 rating methods. J Orthop Sports Phys Ther 2007; 37(3):122–9.
16. Wrigley T, Strauss G. Strength assessment by isokinetic dynamometry. In: Gore CJ, editor. Physiological tests for elite athletes. Champaign (IL): Human Kinetics; 2000. p. 155–99.
17. Wilk KE. Dynamic muscle strength testing. In: Amundsen LR, editor. Muscle strength testing: instrumented and non-instrumented systems. New York: Churchill Livingston; 1990. p. 134–5.
18. Neeter C, Gustavsson A, Thomeé P, et al. Development of a strength test battery for evaluation of leg muscle power after anterior cruciate ligament injury and reconstruction. Knee Surg Sports Traumatol Arthrosc 2006;14:571–680.
19. Greenberger H, Paterno M. Relationship of knee extensor strength and hopping test performance in the assessment of lower extremity function. J Orthop Sports Phys Ther 1995;22:202–6.
20. Pincivero D, Lephart S, Karunakara R. Effects of rest interval on isokinetic strength and functional performance after short-term high intensity training. Br J Sports Med 1997;31:229–34.
21. Pincivero DM, Lephart SM, Karunakara RG. Relation between open and closed kinematic chain assessment of knee strength and functional performance. Clin J Sport Med 1997;7:11–6.
22. Beynnon BD, Johnson RJ, Fleming BC. The science of anterior cruciate ligament rehabilitation. Clin Orthop 2002;402:9–20.
23. Abernethy P, Wilson G, Logan P. Strength and power assessment. Issues, controversies and challenges. Sports Med 1995;19(6):401–17.
24. Daniel DM, Malcolm L, Stone ML, et al. Quantification of knee stability and function. Contemp Orthop 1982;5:83–91.
25. Petsching R, Baron R, Albrecht M. The relationship between isokinetic quadriceps strength test and hop tests for distance and one-legged vertical jump test following anterior cruciate ligament reconstruction. J Orthop Sports Phys Ther 1998;28(1):23–31.
26. Fitzgerald K, Lephart S, Ji Hye Hwang, et al. Hop tests as predictors of dynamic knee stability. J Orthop Sports Phys Ther 2001;31(10):588–97.
27. Bandy W, Rusche K, Tekulve F. Reliability and symmetry for five unilateral functional tests of the lower extremity. Isokinet Exerc Sci 1994;4:108–11.
28. Bolgla L, Keskula D. Reliability of lower extremity functional performance tests. J Orthop Sports Phys Ther 1997;26(3):138–42.
29. Brosky J, Nitz A, Malone TR, et al. Intrarater reliability of selected clinical outcome measures following anterior cruciate ligament reconstruction. J Orthop Sports Phys Ther 1999;29(1):39–48.
30. Eechaute C, Vaes P, Duquet W. Functional performance deficits in patients with CAI: validity of the multiple hop test. Clin J Sport Med 2008;18(2):124–9.
31. Noyes FR, Barber SD, Mangine RE, et al. Quantitative assessment of functional limitations in normal and anterior cruciate ligament deficient knees. Clin Orthop 1990;255:204–14.

32. Reid A, Birmingham B, Stratford PW, et al. Hop testing provides a reliable and valid outcome measure during rehabilitation after cruciate ligament reconstruction. Phys Ther 2007;87(3):337–49.

33. Augustsson J, Thomeé R, Karlsson J. Ability of a new hop test to determine functional deficits after anterior cruciate ligament reconstruction. Knee Surg Sports Traumatol Arthrosc 2004;12:350–6.

34. Gustavsson A, Neeter C, Thomeé P, et al. A test battery for evaluating hop performance in patients with an ACL injury and patients who have undergone ACL reconstruction. Knee Surg Sports Traumatol Arthrosc 2006;14:778–88.

35. Kiesel K, Plisky P, Voight M. Can serious injury in professional football be predicted by a preseason functional movement screen? North American Journal of Sports Physical Therapy 2007;2(3):147–58.

36. Logan P, Fornasiero D, Abernethy P, et al. Protocols for the assessment of isoinertial strength. In: Gore CJ, editor. Physiological tests for elite athletes. Champaign (IL): Human Kinetics; 2000. p. 200–21.

37. Abernethy P, Jürimäe J. Cross-sectional and longitudinal uses of isoinertial, isometric, and isokinetic dynamometry. Med Sci Sports Exerc 1996;28:1180–7.

38. Murphy A, Wilson G, Pryor J. Use of the iso-inertial force mass relationship in the prediction of dynamic human performance. Eur J Appl Physiol 1994;69:250–7.

39. Bompa T. Theory and methodology of training: the key to athletic performance. Dubuque (IA): Kendall Hunt; 1983.

40. Impellizzeri F, Rampinini E, Maffiuletti N, et al. A vertical force jump test for assessing bilateral strength asymmetry in athletes. Med Sci Sports Exerc 2007; 39(11):2044–50.

41. Bangsbo J, Marcello I, Krustrup P. The Yo-Yo intermittent recovery test: a useful tool for evaluation of physical performance in intermittent sports. Sports Med 2008;38(1):37–51.

42. Krustrup P, Mohr M, Ellingsgaard H, et al. Physical demands during an elite female soccer games: importance of training status. Med Sci Sports Exerc 2005;37(7):1242–8.

43. Krustrup P, Mohr M, Amstrup T, et al. The Yo-Yo intermittent recovery test: physiological response, reliability, and validity. Med Sci Sports Exerc 2003;35(4): 697–705.

New Techniques in Articular Cartilage Imaging

Hollis G. Potter, MD*, Brandon R. Black, MD, Le Roy Chong, MD

KEYWORDS

• MRI • Cartilage repair • T2 mapping • T1 rho • dGEMRIC

One of the most important advances in orthopedic imaging over the past 10 years has been the ability to reliably image articular cartilage. Although essential for normal joint function and homeostasis, hyaline cartilage, once injured, has little capacity to undergo spontaneous repair. Early recognition of traumatic chondral injury and early degenerative change permit interventions that are aimed at delaying the progression of osteoarthritis and eventual arthroplasty. Once cartilage repair techniques are performed, new advances in the noninvasive detection of cartilage biochemistry provide insight into the ultrastructure of cartilage repair tissue, eventually obviating the need for surgical biopsy and violation of the repair as well as a providing an objective assessment of treatment outcome.

CARTILAGE STRUCTURE

Hyaline articular cartilage is a viscoelastic substance with strong imaging and biomechanical anisotropy. Articular cartilage has resilience to compression, while transmitting and distributing load, thereby reducing peak stresses on underlying subchondral bone. Joint cartilage also provides a smooth surface and lubrication, permitting the movement of opposing surfaces with minimal friction.[1] Chondrocytes comprise less than 10% of the cartilage volume, with water being the most abundant component. Most of the water is contained within the interstitial space created by the matrix elements. The material properties are attributed to the extracellular matrix elements, with collagen imparting tensile strength and proteoglycan imparting compressive strength.

Matrix composition, organization, mechanical properties, and cell function vary with respect to the depth from the articular surface and result in morphologic differences that allow the identification of 4 layers or zones in articular cartilage. The boundaries between the zones are not sharply defined, but consist of a superficial zone, a transitional zone, a radial zone, and a zone of calcified cartilage (**Fig. 1**).[2]

Magnetic Resonance Imaging, The Hospital for Special Surgery, Weill Medical College of Cornell University, 535 East 70th Street, New York, NY 10021, USA
* Corresponding author. 535 East 70th Street, New York, NY 10021.
E-mail address: potterh@hss.edu (H.G. Potter).

Clin Sports Med 28 (2009) 77–94
doi:10.1016/j.csm.2008.08.004
0278-5919/08/$ – see front matter © 2008 Elsevier Inc. All rights reserved.

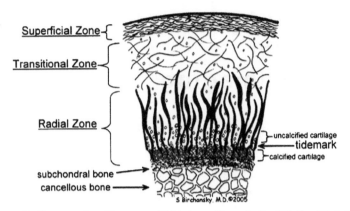

Superficial Zone
Transitional Zone
Radial Zone
uncalcified cartilage
tidemark
calcified cartilage
subchondral bone
cancellous bone
S Birchansky M.D.©2005

Fig.1. Schematic diagram of cartilage zonal histology. (*From* Potter HG, Foo LF. Articular cartilage. In: Stoller DW, editor. Magnetic resonance imaging in orthopaedics and sports medicine. Philadelphia: Lippincott Williams & Wilkins; 2007. p. 1099–130; with permission.)

The thinnest zone, the superficial zone, is subdivided into 2 layers: an acellular surface zone with little proteoglycan known as the lamina splendens, consisting of densely concentrated collagen fibrils oriented parallel to the articular surface, and a deep zone consisting of chondrocytes that express proteins with lubricating and protective functions. These fibrils give this zone greater tensile stiffness and strength than the deeper zones and may resist shear forces generated during use of the joint.[2,3] The transitional zone consists of inhomogeneously oriented collagen fibers, which act to distribute stress more uniformly across loaded tissue.[4] The transitional zone represents 40% to 60% of the cartilage thickness and contains a higher concentration of proteoglycans, but a lower concentration of both collagen and water than the superficial zone. The chondrocytes and collagen fibrils in the radial zone are oriented in columns perpendicular to the articular surface. This zone contains the largest diameter collagen fibrils, the highest concentration of proteoglycans, and the lowest concentration of water. The collagen fibrils of the radial zone pass into the tidemark, which roughly corresponds to the boundary between calcified and uncalcified cartilage. The tidemark also represents a potential shear plane for articular cartilage defects in the adult skeleton.[5,6] The thin zone of calcified cartilage separates the radial zone from the subchondral bone, and the subchondral plate and calcified zone cannot be distinguished as separate structures at clinically relevant field strengths.

MORPHOLOGIC CARTILAGE ASSESSMENT

Although many pulse sequences are suitable for evaluation of articular cartilage, it is important to remember that traditional MRI protocols, including T1- and heavily T2-weighted images, are not effective in assessing articular cartilage. Acceptable accuracy based on an arthroscopic standard and good interobserver variability has been shown using a moderate echo time fast spin-echo sequence in a study of over 600 articular surfaces and 88 patients, generating a weighted Kappa statistic of 0.93, indicating almost perfect agreement.[7] Bredella and colleagues[8] used fat suppression on moderate echo-time imaging and achieved an overall accuracy of 98%.

More recently, 3D techniques with isotropic voxels have become available, allowing for the creation of differential contrast between articular cartilage, fibrocartilage, and fluid, and provide high-resolution isotropic data sets that allow for reformations in orthogonal planes (**Fig. 2**).[9] Many additional gradient-echo pulse sequences are available, which provide contrast between hyaline cartilage, fluid, and fibrocartilage, most of which rely on achieving a steady state, such as balanced steady-state free precession (SSFP), and fluctuating equilibrium magnetic resonance (FEMR). The latter 2 pulse sequences produce a bright signal from fluid with intermediate signal intensity articular cartilage, allowing for the detection of focal surface changes. These techniques may be combined with fat-water separation, such as IDEAL (iterative decomposition of water and fat with echo asymmetry and least-squares estimation), minimizing off-resonance effects.[10]

Data obtained from 3D data sets are suitable for semiautomatic segmentation algorithms, allowing for quantification of cartilage volume over time. It is important to remember, however, that cartilage volume is a function of both thickness and surface area, and longitudinal changes are affected by both alteration in cartilage thickness (areas of cartilage swelling create regions of elevation whereas areas of cartilage thinning create regions of depression) as well as alterations in cartilage surface area (such as the development of osteophyte formation).[11] Cicuttini and colleagues[12] compared tibial cartilage volume to radiographs in a group of over 250 patients,

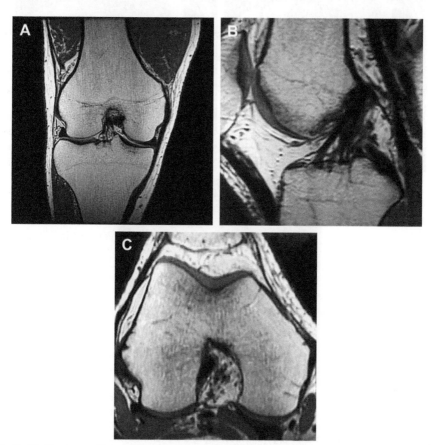

Fig. 2. (*A–C*) Intermediate-weighted MR image (*A*) of the knee in a 35-year-old healthy volunteer acquired using a volumetric extended echo train acquisition (XETA) prescribed in the coronal plane; the data set generates near-isotropic voxels, which may be manipulated in various planes, in this instance, allowing for high-resolution reformations in the sagittal (*B*) and axial (*C*) planes.

demonstrating a strong negative linear association between the tibial cartilage volume and the increasing grade of joint space narrowing.[12] The correlation was strengthened when values were adjusted for age, gender, and body mass index. Conversely, Raynauld and colleagues[13] studied 32 patients with symptomatic knee osteoarthritis using MRI and noted no statistical correlation between loss of cartilage volume and radiographic changes, demonstrating the relative insensitivity of traditional weight-bearing radiographs in the longitudinal assessment of osteoarthritis.

Despite these challenges, 3D models of cartilage will likely prove useful in the future development of tissue engineering techniques. Using projection algorithms that are color-coded for thickness will allow detection of regional alterations in cartilage morphology, when planning for potential focal surface or complete joint resurfacing procedures (**Fig. 3**).

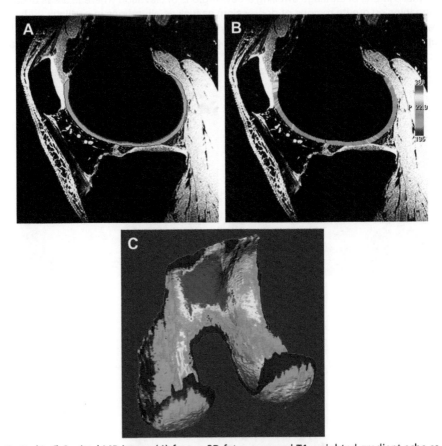

Fig. 3. (*A–C*) Sagittal MR image (*A*) from a 3D fat-suppressed T1-weighted gradient echo sequence of the knee in a 35-year-old healthy volunteer. The reconstructed images from the volumetric data show high cartilage–bone contrast and can be manipulated in various planes, thus ideal for cartilage segmentation using a signal-intensity-based semiautomated algorithm. Color map (*B*) generated from the segmentation data shows regional cartilage thickness distribution, with the blue end of the scale coded for areas of relatively thinner cartilage and the red end of the scale for areas of relatively thicker cartilage. 3D rendered model (*C*) of the articular cartilage from the segmentation data has been color-coded to reflect regional thickness distribution using a similar scale as in (*B*).

MRI ASSESSMENT OF CARTILAGE ULTRASTRUCTURE: PROTEOGLYCAN
Delayed Gadolinium-Enhanced MRI of Cartilage

The compressive strength of the proteoglycans is understood when one notes that the proteoglycan monomers, with their negatively charged glycosaminoglycans (GAG; chondroitin sulfate or keratin sulfate), radiate from a protein core. These monomers bind to hyaluronic acid to form large aggregates that resist compression due to their highly hydrophilic structure. Strategies that are sensitive to the proteoglycan component of the extracellular matrix may exploit the negative fixed-charge of the GAG constituents, thereby assessing fixed-charge density. Techniques used to assess proteoglycan include sodium (Na^{23}) imaging, dGEMRIC, and T1rho (T1ρ) imaging. Sodium imaging in clinical systems of field strengths of 3 T or lower is limited by the relatively decreased abundance of sodium in articular cartilage compared with hydrogen, reducing the signal-to-noise ratio and requiring long scan times. It also requires specialty coils and the ability to scan with multinuclear spectroscopy software, which is not widely available across clinical systems.

Delayed dGEMRIC techniques require a double dose of an intravenous, negatively charged, gadolinium salt (Gd-DTPA). Following a brief period of exercise (approximately 10 minutes) followed by a 90-minute delay, scanning is performed, typically using a two-dimensional fast inversion recovery technique. As gadolinium acts to shorten T1 relaxation time, one may generate T1 maps that display, on a pixel-by-pixel basis, the T1 relaxation time within the cartilage voxel being studied. Following injection, the contrast agent will penetrate into the cartilage, providing an index of regional gadolinium concentration in the cartilage, which is in turn related to the glycosaminoglycan concentration in the tissue (**Fig. 4**).[14,15]

The ability to noninvasively detect depletion of matrix elements has proven useful in the early detection of osteoarthritis. Such tools will be helpful in determining the optimal timing of surgical procedures that are aimed at delaying the progression of osteoarthritis, such as osteotomy and meniscal transplantation. In a study of patients with

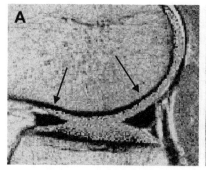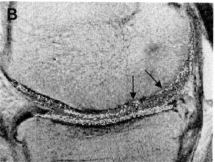

Fig. 4. (*A–B*) Global and focal ranges of glycosaminoglycan distribution (T1$_{Gd}$) index. Sagittal T1$_{Gd}$ MR image (*A*) of the lateral compartment in a 26-year-old female professional dancer shows high-range (blue–green areas) T1$_{Gd}$ values (mean ± SD, 547 ± 121 ms) of the tibial plateau and weight-bearing zones of the femoral condyle (*arrows*). Sagittal T1$_{Gd}$ MR image (*B*) from a 78-year-old woman with moderately severe medial osteoarthritis reveals T1$_{Gd}$ values in low range (*red areas*) (285 ± 74 ms) for the medial femoral condyle with focal areas (*arrows*) displaying lower values (243 ± 56 ms). Mean T1$_{Gd}$ index of the surrounding cartilage was 312 ± 75 ms. (*From* Williams A, Gillis A, McKenzie C, et al. Glycosaminoglycan distribution in cartilage as determined by dGEMRIC: potential clinical applications. AJR Am J Roentgenol 2004;182:167–72; with permission.)

developmental dysplasia of the hip, the dGEMRIC index was found to be sensitive to arthritis changes as well as symptoms (assessed by the Western Ontario and McMaster Universities Osteoarthritis (WOMAC) questionnaire) and correlated to the severity of dysplasia, as assessed on conventional radiographs by measuring the lateral center-edge angle.[16] In this study, radiographs did not correlate to pain scores.[16] In a subsequent follow-up study of patients with dysplasia treated with osteotomy, those with osteotomy failures had more arthritis on radiographs as well as lower dGEMRIC indices, indicating greater depletion of proteoglycans; further analysis indicated that the dGEMRIC index was the most important predictor of osteotomy failure.[17] The investigators concluded that these MRI techniques may prove helpful in identifying suitable candidates for pelvic osteotomy.

T1rho (T1ρ) Imaging

T1ρ is a technique that has been used to assess low-frequency interactions between hydrogen and macromolecules in free water. It is termed spin lattice relaxation in the rotating frame, using clusters of radiofrequency pulses to "lock" magnetization in the transverse plane, followed by additional radiofrequency pulses to drive longitudinal recovery. Capturing several values allows one to solve for the slope of the decay function and create either gray-scale or color-coded maps (**Fig. 5**). Previous validation of T1ρ has been performed at multiple field strengths. T1ρ has been shown to correlate to proteoglycan content and fixed charge density in both enzymatically degraded bovine and clinical osteoarthritis specimens at 4 T.[18] The investigators compared normalized T1ρ rate (1/T1ρ), standardized as a percent change from normal cartilage, to assessment of fixed charge density from Na^{23} and to histology, using alcian blue-periodic acid-Schiff (PAS) staining.[18] The percentage change of T1ρ and fixed charge density was highly correlated (R^2 value> 0.75 and 0.85; $P < 0.001$) and T1ρ values were found to increase as proteoglycan concentrations decreased.[18] An additional study at 4 T used an in vivo porcine model of rapidly induced cytokine-mediated cartilage degeneration through the intra-articular injection of recombinant interleukin-1β (IL-1β), to induce changes in cartilage by way of matrix metalloprotease induction.[19] In this non-clinical model of osteoarthritis, the investigators correlated the T1ρ imaging results with histology and immunohistochemical staining. A strong correlation coefficient was found between in vivo and ex vivo data ($R^2 = 0.86$; $P < 0.001$), and proteoglycan loss was seen by histologic staining as well as decreased Na concentration.[19]

Li and colleagues[20] have shown the clinical feasibility of T1ρ at 3 T and studied both T1ρ and T2 relaxation times in clinical volunteers. The investigators noted that where a significant correlation was found between T1ρ and T2, the difference of T2 was not significant between controls and osteoarthritic patients, suggesting that T1ρ may be more sensitive in early degenerative changes in cartilage. The latter finding is not surprising, as one would anticipate that the proteoglycan depletion precedes that of disruption of collagen in the setting of early osteoarthritis.

MRI ASSESSMENT OF CARTILAGE ULTRASTRUCTURE: COLLAGEN
T2 Mapping

One of the strategies to assess the collagen component of articular cartilage is T2 mapping. The collagen fibers within type-1 collagen provide tensile strength due to their high ratio of length to thickness. Both intramolecular and intermolecular cross-linking provide structural rigidity to the collagen fibrils and prevent slipping and sliding between the collagen molecules. This highly ordered structure, when bound with water, provides the important network for maintaining part of the cartilage structural

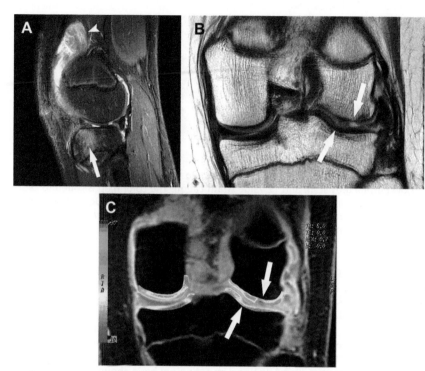

Fig. 5. (*A–C*) Sagittal fat-suppressed (*A*) and coronal (*B*) fast spin-echo MR images from the knee in a 15 year-old girl following subtotal lateral meniscectomy 3 mo prior reveals marked synovitis (*arrowhead*) in response to active cartilage delamination (*B, arrows*) from the lateral femoral condyle and plateau, with edema and focal subchondral fracture (*A, arrow*). Coronal T1ρ map (*C*) shows corresponding areas of prolonged T1ρ values in the lateral femoral condyle and tibial plateau, indicative of areas of proteoglycan depletion. The color map is coded to capture T1ρ values ranging from 10 to 90 ms, with green reflecting longer values; yellow, intermediate values; and orange/red, shorter values.

integrity. There is also a very highly ordered arrangement of collagen within the articular cartilage. Within the deep radial zone, collagen is oriented perpendicular to the subchondral plate. The vertical striation of this cartilage may be evident on clinical MRI, and the basilar components typically have shorter T2 values (**Fig. 6**). In the transitional zone, collagen is more randomly oriented and has longer T2 values. The superficial zone, depending on the spatial resolution of the clinical MRI parameters, may be beyond the spatial resolution of the technique but may be perceived as a thin, hypointense line of additionally ordered collagen, this time parallel to the subchondral bone (**Fig. 7**).

T2 mapping is the pixel-by-pixel solving of the T2 relaxation curve. T2 relaxation is an exponential decay function that reflects the loss of signal that occurs rapidly as a function in time due the dephasing of the excited nuclei after the disturbing radiofrequency pulse is applied. Tissues that maintain internuclear phase coherence and, therefore, decay more slowly can demonstrate a signal that is perceptible on clinical MRI and may be quantified using appropriate MR pulse sequences to perform T2 mapping. In contrast, some substances decay very rapidly and thus have very short T2 relaxation times that preclude their measurement on standard MR sequences.

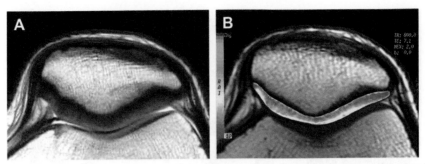

Fig. 6. (*A–B*) Axial fast spin-echo (*A*) and T2 relaxation time color map (*B*) from a 27-year-old man show normal gray scale and T2 value stratification. The color map is coded to capture T2 values ranging from 10 to 90 ms, with green reflecting longer T2 values; yellow, intermediate values; and orange/red, shorter values. Stratification of T2 values with shorter values is seen in the radial zone, where water is most restricted.

To obtain a signal from very short T2 species, such as the type-1 collagen of tendons, ligaments, menisci and the basilar components of cartilage, including the calcified zone, specialized pulse sequences known as ultrashort echo time techniques (UTE) are necessary (**Figs. 8, 9**).[21,22]

The orientational alignment of articular cartilage may be visualized using color-coded T2 maps. The T2 characteristics of cartilage have been shown to be statistically equivalent to the histologic zones of collagen fibril orientation, using polarized light microscopy as the standard.[23,24] Additional investigators have shown that proteoglycan depletion has little effect on the T2 of cartilage,[25] and Mlynárik and colleagues[26] found no difference in quantitative T2 values between normal and enzymatically depleted areas of proteoglycan loss, noted in human explant cartilage.

T2 relaxation time is influenced by the structural anisotropy of the collagen. There is a well-defined relationship between the excited hydrogen dipoles within the collagen and the long axis of the magnetic field, which in the traditional closed MR unit runs parallel to the long axis of the patient's body. When the angle between the external field and the spinning hydrogen nuclei reaches approximately 55°, there is an expected

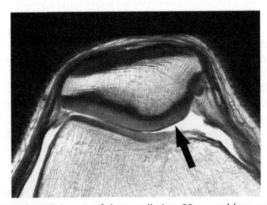

Fig. 7. Axial fast spin-echo MR image of the patella in a 39-year-old man shows a thin, hypointense line over the articular surface of the patella (*arrow*), representing the superficial zone of the cartilage (lamina splendens).

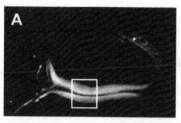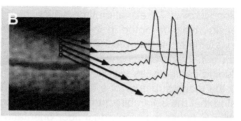

Fig. 8. (*A–B*) Axial MR images of the patellofemoral joint of a 25-year-old healthy volunteer using projection–reconstruction spectroscopic imaging sequence (TE = 200 ms). (*A*) Water-frequency image. (*B*) Magnified image of articular cartilage from box in (*A*), along with spectra of patellofemoral cartilage. Note the decreasing line width and increasing peak area as voxels progress from the cartilage–bone interface to articular surface. (*From* Gold GE, Thedens DR, Pauly JM, et al. MR imaging of articular cartilage of the knee: new methods using ultrashort TEs. AJR Am J Roentgenol 1998;170:1223–6; with permission.)

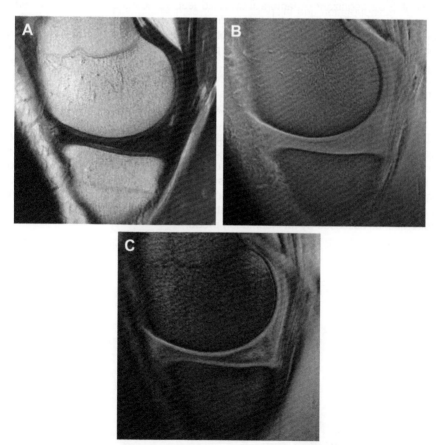

Fig. 9. Sagittal fast spin-echo (*A*) and ultra-short TE sequence (UTE) MR images (*B, C*) from the medial knee compartment in a healthy 35-year-old volunteer. The images were acquired at echo times of 25 ms, 0.3 ms, and 5.8 ms, respectively. The fast spin-echo image shows paucity of signal arising from the meniscus, with intrasubstance signal generated on the UTE images; this is related to the very short T2 relaxation time of meniscal fibrocartilage and the echo times used.

prolongation of T2 relaxation time, which is clinically manifested as increased signal intensity, typically noted in the basilar components of the articular cartilage where the water is most restricted (**Fig. 10**). Although attributed by some to an artifact, this is an expected relationship between the highly ordered structure of soft tissues, including cartilage, as well as tendons and ligaments.[27,28] Providing greater insight into the macrostructure of articular cartilage, Goodwin and colleagues[29] have suggested that the 3D architecture and regional variations in the arrangement of articular cartilage, rather than individual fiber orientation, may account for alterations in the appearance noted on clinical MR images as well as quantitative T2 maps. This is particularly in light of the fact that in clinical MR imaging, one creates individual slices that will not necessarily sample cartilage tangential to the subchondral plate throughout the slice, creating partial volume sampling effects. This could account for areas of regional T2 variation, for example, in the submeniscal zone of the tibia compared with the contral zone (**Fig. 11**).

In addition to an awareness of the 3D architecture of the extracellular matrix, one must also be cognizant of factors that could lead to sources of quantitative error when performing T1 or T2 mapping, including receiver coil, parameter selection, signal-to-noise ratio, and voxel size. Control for these sources of error may require code modification, and standardization of protocols and quantitative methodologies is essential before initiating a multisite trial that uses quantitative MRI as an outcome measure.[30] More efficient quantification of relaxation times may be performed using parallel imaging, which uses spatial encoding from individual coil elements of the receiver array to reduce encoding steps and thereby accelerate data acquisition.[31]

Prolonged T2 relaxation time is associated with osteoarthritis and breakdown of cartilage architecture.[32–34] Kelly and colleagues[35] provided supporting evidence in an ovine meniscectomy model of osteoarthritis; the investigators showed that prolonged T2 values observed following meniscectomy correlated to degradation of collagen as assessed by the Mankin scale on polarized light microscopy. In the same study, prolonged T2 also correlated strongly to alterations in biomechanical properties, as assessed by an indentation probe.[35]

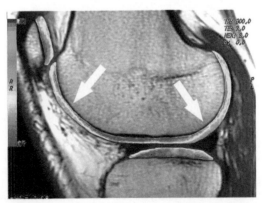

Fig. 10. Sagittal T2 map from the knee in a 25-year-old woman shows prolongation of T2 values (*arrows*) in the anterior and posterior aspects of the lateral femoral condyle related to magic angle phenomenon, caused by the structural anisotropy of collagen relative to the static magnetic field.

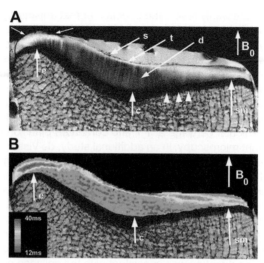

Fig. 11. (*A–B*) Lateral tibial plateau of a 35-year-old woman. B_0 = main magnetic field. On mid-coronal (*A*) spin-echo image (TR/TE, 1,000/14; field of view, 45 mm; slice thickness, 1 mm; matrix size, 512 × 512), variations in signal intensity produce a characteristic three-layered appearance. In the central region of the plateau (c), in which a higher-signal-intensity transitional layer (t) is thin, and radial striations extend across thick deep layer (d), and minor fibrillation is seen at the low-signal-intensity surface (s). In the submeniscal region (sm) and at the tibial eminence (e), the transitional layer is much thicker. Chemical shift produces a low-signal-intensity interface at the subchondral bone (*arrowheads*). Surface of tibial eminence (*short arrows*) does not interface with saline and cannot be clearly visualized because of contact of wax enclosure with the joint surface. On the corresponding T2 map (*B*), changes in T2 parallel changes in signal intensity. Peak T2 values are located in middle of transitional layer. c, central region of plateau; e, tibial eminence; sm, submeniscal region. (*From* Goodwin DW, Wadghiri YZ, Zhu H, et al. Macroscopic structure of articular cartilage of the tibial plateau: influence of a characteristic matrix architecture on MRI appearance. AJR Am J Roentgenol 2004;182:311–8; with permission.)

Diffusion-Weighted Imaging and Diffusion Tensor Imaging

DWI has long been used in neuroimaging for the detection of early ischemia, which is manifested as focal restriction in the diffusion of water. Given the high water content of articular cartilage, these techniques have been recently applied as markers of structural integrity of cartilage. The background of DWI entails the addition of diffusion weighting to an MR pulse sequence, using a pair of gradients with opposite polarity, the effect of which creates attenuation of signal due to dispersion of spins. The amount of signal reduction is proportional to the amount of diffusion in the tissue and can be measured as an apparent diffusion coefficient (ADC). Local diffusivity in any soft tissue can be defined as a vector quantity with a magnitude and direction; these are in the direction of the macromolecular environment of the tissue being imaged. Thus, in a clinical joint, free water demonstrates unrestricted diffusion, whereas bound water demonstrates "spatially restricted diffusivity."[36,37] Investigators have demonstrated a gradual decrease in apparent diffusion coefficient values from the surface down to the tidemark.[36]

With the use of several diffusion-sensitive gradient pairs in non-coplanar directions, DTI has the ability to provide directional information with regard to the thickness of cartilage. Whereas quantitative T2 measurements reflect the structural anisotropy of tissue, they do not necessarily reflect the direction of that anisotropy. The addition of these multiple diffusion sensitizing gradient pairs placed in different directions allows DTI to provide a symmetric matrix, reporting a pixel-specific component of the diffusion pathway, known as the diffusion tensor.[38] The 3 main directions of diffusion correspond to the 3 main axes of anisotropy, the so-called "eigenvectors," with their absolute values reflecting the eigenvalue of the tensor.[36]

In articular cartilage, DTI has been shown to be sensitive to the direction of the collagen component of the extracellular matrix.[39–42] De Visser and colleagues[42] studied samples of bovine articular cartilage at 7 T and correlated diffusion tensor alignment ngles to polarized light microscopy. In an additional study, de Visser and colleagues[41] correlated compressive strain applied to bovine explants at 7 T and discerned that compression resulted in a decrease in both the maximum and mean eigenvalues, with a change in the average orientation of the principal eigenvalue, indicating that tho collagen response to the compressive load was to orient more parallel to the surface. These experiments provide insight into tho structural changes in the alignment of the collagen network during simulated function and loading condition. Evaluating human femoral cartilage bone explants at 8.45 T, Deng and colleagues[37] noted that the measured diffusion direction was consistent with the collagen network. Following trypsin degradation of the samples with associated GAG loss, there was little to no change in the diffusion anisotropy, suggesting that collagen had the predominant influence on the direction of water diffusion in hyaline cartilage.

Although these data are still preliminary, DTI may become a powerful tool in the noninvasive study of cartilage structure and function and may provide insight into changes observed as a result of degradation in the setting of osteoarthritis or traumatic chondral injury. At clinically relevant field strengths and clinical systems, challenges in DWI include sensitivity to motion artifact and requirement of echo times sufficiently short enough to maximize cartilage signal as well as imaging strategies that act to improve the signal-to-noise ratio. Despite these challenges, images that demonstrate fractional anisotropy may be obtained and provide insight into orientation of the collagen (**Fig. 12**). DWI and DTI are promising techniques to visualize cartilage ultrastructure.

LINKING MRI TO CARTILAGE MATERIAL PROPERTIES

Additional focus will be placed on linking quantitative MR assessment to material properties. The in vitro study of human patellar cartilage samples by T2 mapping and dGEMRIC measures were made at both 1.5 T and 9.4 T and were then correlated with static and dynamic compressive moduli at 6 discrete anatomic locations.[43] It is worth noting that statistically significant linear correlations were observed between T2 mapping and mechanical properties at clinically relevant field strength, suggesting that T2 may provide indirect insight into material properties.[43] At a microscopic-level field strength of 8.45 T, Samosky and colleagues[44] noted that the dGEMRIC index of tibial explants correlated to local stiffness when the GAG index was normalized to the depth of the indented tissue, but not for the full thickness of the GAG index, thereby concluding that other factors may contribute to focal alterations in indentation stiffness. Dynamic MR elastography has more recently been proposed as a method for the noninvasive assessment of mechanical properties of biologic soft tissues. Using motion-sensitive phase contrast MR methods and specialized gradients that detect shear deformations, images obtained reflect a time frame of cyclical shear deformation of tissue as it propagates throughout the media studied.[45] Appropriately applied algorithms then allow for the calculation of internal distribution of shear stiffness within

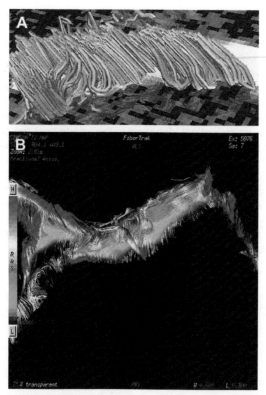

Fig. 12. (A–B) Diffusion tensor image (A) with fiber tracking of a bovine cartilage sample at 3 T. DTI (B) of cartilage color-coded according to fractional anisotropy. The color map is coded to reflect regional anisotropy, with green indicating areas of less restricted and orange/red areas of more restricted diffusion.

the tissue from the physical displacement measurement obtained on the phase images.[45,46] In the former study, the investigators are able to demonstrate high-resolution shear stiffness measurements of hyaline cartilage using a special gradient coil system, which allows superior gradient performance, beyond the capabilities of a traditional 1.5 T clinical scanner.[45] Although these techniques remain challenging, the development of capabilities by which to link MR data with material properties is warranted and may eventually provide predictive information concerning the durability of tissue engineered constructs and cartilage repair.

MRI ASSESSMENT OF CARTILAGE REPAIR

MRI provides an essential objective outcome standard to augment the information obtained from validated subjective outcome instruments, such as pain and function scores. Given the limited ability of articular cartilage to undergo primary repair, many surgical procedures have been developed to repair tissue, including marrow stimulation techniques such as microfracture, osteochondral transfer using either autologous or allograft tissue, and tissue engineered techniques, which require a matrix scaffold (either carbohydrate-based polymers or protein-based polymers such as collagen), cells (chondrocytes, chondroprogenitor cell pools, or mesenchymal stem cells), and signaling molecules (**Fig. 13**).

In an observational study of 112 patients (180 MRI examinations), of autologous cartilage implantation (ACI) and microfracture, Brown and colleagues[47] defined several variables that proved effective in the assessment of cartilage repair morphology, including (1) the relative signal intensity from the repaired area compared with native cartilage using a standardized region of interest (ROI) analysis; (2) the morphology of repair (flush, depressed, or proud) with respect to the adjacent cartilage; (3) the presence or absence of delamination; (4) nature of the interface at the edge of peripheral integration; (5) the percentage of fill based on both the coronal and sagittal images; (6) assessment at the adjacent and opposite cartilage; (7) any adverse synovial response. Compared with microfracture, ACI demonstrated consistently better fill at all times but was complicated by the presence of graft hypertrophy in almost two-thirds (19/30) of repairs and was most commonly seen in the initial 6-month follow-up period. The signal characteristics of the repair tissue were generally hyperintense to that of hyaline cartilage at short term (less than 6 months) follow-up, with progressive maturation over time, particularly in the ACI group.[47]

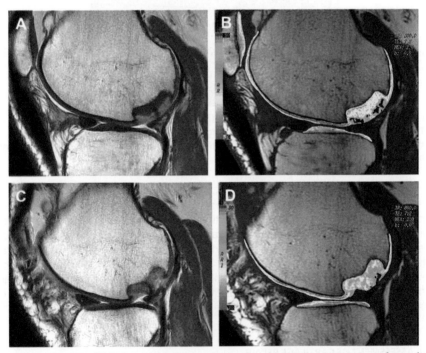

Fig. 13. (A–D) Sagittal fast spin-echo MR images and corresponding T2 maps performed at 6 mo (A, B) and 12 mo (C, D) in a 54 year-old woman following synthetic acellular biphasic copolymer plugs insertion into the lateral femoral condyle. Compared with the 6-month study, MRI at 12 mo shows interval progressive but incomplete osseous incorporation of the bone phase of the plugs, with depression of the articular surfaces and diminished fill of the articular phase of the plugs. There is marked T2 prolongation over both the articular and osseous phases of the plugs, which is an expected finding at 12 months follow-up. The color maps are coded to capture T2 values ranging from 10 to 90 ms, with green reflecting longer T2 values; yellow, intermediate values; and orange/red, shorter values.

Marlovits and colleagues[48] defined an MRI observation of cartilage repair tissue (MOCART) using similar variables and assessed 13 patients at 24 months follow-up. The investigators evaluated 9 parameters, including the degree of fill and integration of the defect, the structure, surface integrity, and signal intensity of the repair tissue, the integrity of the subchondral lamina and bone, and the presence of "adhesions" and/or effusion. It is worth noting, the investigators correlated to the knee injury and osteoarthritis outcome score (KOOS) and visual analog score (VAS) for pain and function and noted that clinical scores were correlated to several of the MRI variables, finding significant correlation for amount of fill, structure of the repair tissue, changes in the subchondral bone, and signal intensity of the repair tissue. Further, intraclass correlation coefficients (ICC) were performed and ranged between 0.76 and 1.00, indicating strong agreement between observers.[48]

Welsch and colleagues[49] prospectively compared T2 mapping of microfracture to matrix-associated autologous chondrocyte transplantation (MACT) with a mean follow-up of 28.6 and 27.4 months for microfracture and MACT, respectively. The investigators noted that in the microfracture group, the mean T2 was significantly reduced relative to native cartilage ($P < 0.05$) when compared with MACT. With regard to the assessment of zonal stratification of T2 similar to that of hyaline cartilage, microfracture repair demonstrated no significant trend as a function of repair depth, whereas MACT showed a significant increase in mean T2 values from deep to superficial zones ($P < 0.05$).[49]

Gillis and colleagues[50] evaluated ACI with dGEMRIC techniques and studied 11 implants at 2- to 24-month intervals, finding that the relative GAG index in grafts implanted for less than 12 months was lower than that of native cartilage, whereas those studied at longer than 12 months follow-up demonstrated GAG indices that were comparable to native cartilage.

In another prospective study of 48 patients treated with microfracture evaluated by validated clinical outcome instruments and cartilage-sensitive MRI, Mithoefer and colleagues[51] noted that adverse functional scores after 24 months correlated with poor percentage fill. The prospective studies, in particular, demonstrate the effectiveness of MRI in providing objective assessment of cartilage repair and that certain variables correlate to clinical outcome.

With regard to osteochondral transfer, Williams and colleagues[52] performed a prospective longitudinal study of cartilage defects treated with hypothermically stored fresh osteochondral allografts using validated clinical outcome instruments and MRI. Fissures were noted at the graft–host interface in 84% (16/19) of grafts and poor incorporation was noted in 32% (6/19) of grafts, 3 of which had intense bone marrow edema and 3 had frank subchondral marrow fibrosis, manifested as low signal on all pulse sequences. Collapse of the subchondral bone in the graft was correlated to the lack of bony integration based on signal characteristics, indicating that MRI may be predictive of eventual allograft failure.[52] Sirlin and colleagues[53] correlated MRI of shell osteochondral allografts to the results of antihuman leukocyte antigen–antibody screening. In the latter study, patients who expressed positive humoral immune responses were associated with decreased graft incorporation, more intense bone marrow edema pattern, and a higher proportion of surface collapse of the graft.[53]

SUMMARY

Standardized MRI pulse sequences are now readily available and provide an accurate, reproducible assessment of cartilage morphology. 3D modeling techniques enable semiautomated models of the joint surface, which may eventually prove essential in templating before partial or total joint resurfacing. The addition of quantitative MRI techniques provides insights into tissue biochemistry in a noninvasive fashion, and the link to material properties may predict the functional capacity of native and repaired tissue. MRI provides an essential objective assessment of cartilage regenerative procedures.

REFERENCES

1. Mow VC, Proctor CS, Kelly MA. Biomechanics of articular cartilage. In: Nordin M, Frankel VH, editors. Basic biomechanics of tissues and structure of the musculo-skeletal system. Philadelphia: Lea & Febiger; 1989. p. 31–58.
2. Roth V, Mow VC. The intrinsic tensile behavior of the matrix of bovine articular car-tilage and its variation with age. J Bone Joint Surg Am 1980;62:1102–17.
3. Mow VC, Rosenwasser MP. Articular cartilage biomechanics. Injury and repair of the musculoskeletal soft tissues. Park Ridge, IL: The American Academy of Orthopedic Surgeons; 1988. p. 427–63.
4. Askew MJ, Mow VC. The biomechanical function of the collagen ultrastructure of articular cartilage. J Biomech Eng 1978;100:105–15.
5. Bullough PG, Jagannath A. The morphology of the calcification front in articular cartilage. Its significance in joint function. J Bone Joint Surg Br 1983;65:72–8.
6. Bullough PG, Goodfellow J. The significance of the fine structure of articular car-tilage. J Bone Joint Surg Br 1968;50:852–7.
7. Potter HG, Linklater JA, Allen AA, et al. Magnetic resonance imaging of articular cartilage in the knee: an evaluation with use of fast spin-echo imaging. J Bone Joint Surg Am 1998;80:1276–84.
8. Bredella MA, Tirman PF, Peterfy CG, et al. Accuracy of T2-weighted fast spin echo MR imaging with fat saturation in detecting cartilage defects in the knee: comparison with arthroscopy in 130 patients. AJR Am J Roentgenol 1999;172: 1073–80.
9. Gold GE, Busse RE, Beehler C, et al. Isotopic MRI of the knee with 3D fast spin-echo extended echo-train acquisition (XETA): initial experience. AJR 2007;188: 1287–93.
10. Gold GE, Burstein D, Dardzinski B, et al. MRI of articular cartilage in OA: novel pulse sequences and compositional/functional markers. Osteoarthr Cartil 2006; 14:A76–86.
11. Eckstein F, Glaser C. Measuring cartilage morphology with quantitative magnetic resonance imaging. Semin Musculoskelet Radiol 2004;8:329–53.
12. Cicuttini FM, Wluka AE, Forbes A, et al. Comparison of tibial cartilage volume and radiologic grade of the tibiofemoral joint. Arthritis Rheum 2003;48:682–8.
13. Raynauld JP, Martel-Pelletier J, Berthiaume MJ, et al. Quantitative magnetic res-onance imaging evaluation of knee osteoarthritis progression over two years and correlation with clinical symptoms and radiologic changes. Arthritis Rheum 2004; 50:476–87.
14. Bashir A, Gray ML, Boutin RD, et al. Glycosaminoglycan in articular cartilage: in vivo assessment with delayed Gd (DTPA)$^{2-}$ -enhanced MR imaging. Radiology 1997;205:551–8.
15. Williams A, Gillis A, McKenzie C, et al. Glycosaminoglycan distribution in carti-lage as determined by delayed gadolinium-enhanced MRI of cartilage (dGEM-RIC): potential clinical applications. AJR 2004;182:167–72.
16. Kim YJ, Jaramillo D, Millis MB, et al. Assessment of early osteoarthritis in hip dys-plasia with delayed gadolinium-enhanced magnetic resonance imaging of carti-lage. J Bone Joint Surg 2003;85A:1987–92.

17. Cunningham T, Jessel R, Zurakowski D, et al. Delayed gadolinium-enhanced magnetic resonance imaging of cartilage to predict early failure of Bernese periacetabular osteotomy for hip dysplasia. J Bone Joint Surg Am 2006;88: 1540–8.
18. Wheaton AJ, Casey FL, Gougoutas AJ, et al. Correlation of $T_{1\rho}$ with fixed charge density in cartilage. J Magn Reson Imaging 2004;20:519–25.
19. Wheaton AJ, Dodge GR, Borthakur A, et al. Detection of changes in articular cartilage proteoglycan by T1ρ magnetic resonance imaging. J Orthop Res 2005;23: 102–8.
20. Li X, Han ET, Ma CB, et al. In vivo 3T spiral imaging based multislice $T_{1\rho}$ mapping of knee cartilage in osteoarthritis. Magn Reson Med 2005;54:929–36.
21. Benjamin M, Bydder GJM. Magnetic resonance imaging of entheses using ultrashort TE (UTE) pulse sequences. J Magn Reson Imaging 2007;25:381–9.
22. Gold GE, Thedens DR, Pauly JM, et al. MR imaging of articular cartilage of the knee: new methods using ultrashort TEs. AJR 1998;170:1223–6.
23. Xia Y, Moody JB, Burton-Wurster N, et al. Quantitative in situ correlation between microscopic MRI and polarized light microscopy studies of articular cartilage. Osteoarthr Cartil 2001;9:393–406.
24. Nieminen MT, Rieppo J, Töyräs J, et al. T2 relaxation reveals spatial collagen architecture in articular cartilage: a comparative quantitative MRI and polarized light microscopic study. Magn Reson Med 2001;26:487–93.
25. Borthakur A, Shapiro EM, Beers J, et al. Sensitivity of MRI to proteoglycan depletion in cartilage: comparison of sodium and proton MRI. Osteoarthr Cartil 2000;8: 288–93.
26. Mlynárik V, Trattnig S, Huber M, et al. The role of relaxation times in monitoring proteoglycan depletion in articular cartilage. J Magn Reson Imaging 1999;10:497–502.
27. Xia Y. Relaxation anisotropy in cartilage by NMR microscopy (μMRI) at 14-μm resolution. Magn Reson Med 1998;39:941–9.
28. Bydder M, Rahal A, Fullerton GD, et al. The magic angle effect: a source of artifact, determinant of image contrast, and technique for imaging. J Magn Reson Imaging 2007;25:290–300.
29. Goodwin DW, Wadghiri YZ, Zhu H, et al. Macroscopic structure of articular cartilage of the tibial plateau: influence of a characteristic matrix architecture on MRI appearance. AJR 2004;182:311–8.
30. Maier CF, Tan SG, Hariharan H, et al. T_2 quantitation of articular cartilage at 1.5 T. J Magn Reson Imaging 2003;17:358–64.
31. Zuo J, Li X, Banerjee S, et al. Parallel imaging of knee cartilage at 3 Tesla. J Magn Reson Imaging 2007;26:1001–9.
32. David-Vaudey E, Ghosh S, Ries M, et al. T2 relaxation time measurements in osteoarthritis. Magn Reson Imaging 2004;22:673–82.
33. Alhadlaq HA, Xia Y, Moody JB, et al. Detecting structural changes in early experimental osteoarthritis of tibial cartilage by microscopic magnetic resonance imaging and polarized light microscopy. Ann Rheum Dis 2004;63:709–17.
34. Mosher TJ, Dardzinski BJ, Smith MB. Human articular cartilage: influence of aging and early symptomatic degeneration on the spatial variation of T2: preliminary findings at 3T. Radiology 2000;214:259–66.
35. Kelly BT, Potter HG, Deng X, et al. Meniscal allograft transplantation in the sheep knee: evaluation of chondroprotective effects. Am J Sports Med 2006;34: 1464–77.
36. Glaser C. New techniques for cartilage imaging: T2 relaxation time and diffusion-weighted MR imaging. Radiol Clin North Am 2005;43:641–53.

37. Deng X, Farley M, Nieminen MT, et al. Diffusion tensor imaging of native and degenerated human articular cartilage. Magn Reson Imaging 2007;25:168–71.
38. Le Bihan D, Mangin JF, Poupon C, et al. Diffusion tensor imaging: concepts and applications. J Magn Reson Imaging 2001;14:534–46.
39. Meder R, de Visser SK, Bowden JC, et al. Diffusion tensor imaging of articular cartilage as a measure of tissue microstructure. Osteoarthr Cartil 2006;14: 875–81.
40. Filidoro L, Dietrich O, Weber J, et al. High-resolution diffusion tensor imaging of human patellar cartilage: feasibility and preliminary findings. Magn Reson Med 2005;53:993–8.
41. de Visser SK, Crawford RW, Pope JM. Structural adaptations in compressed articular cartilage measured by diffusion tensor imaging. Osteoarthr Cartil 2008;16:83–9.
42. de Visser SK, Bowden JC, Wontrup Byrne E, et al. Anisotropy of collagen fibre alignment in bovine cartilage: comparison of polarized light microscopy and spatially resolved diffusion-tensor measurements. Osteoarthritis Cartilage 2008; 16(6):689–97.
43. Lammentausta E, Kiviranta P, Nissi MJ, et al. T2 relaxation time and delayed gadolinium-enhanced MRI of cartilage (dGEMRIC) of human patellar cartilage at 1.5 T and 9.4 T: relationships with tissue mechanical properties. J Orthop Res 2006;24:366–74.
44. Samosky JT, Burstein D, Grimson WE, et al. Spatially-localized correlation of dGEMRIC-measured GAG distribution and mechanical stiffness in the human tibial plateau. J Orthop Res 2005;23:93–101.
45. Lopez O, Amrami KK, Manduca A, et al. Developments in dynamic MR elastography for in vitro biomechanical assessment of hyaline cartilage under high-frequency cyclical shear. J Magn Reson Imaging 2007;25:310–20.
46. Manduca A, Oliphant TE, Dresner MA, et al. Magnetic resonance elastography: non-invasive mapping of tissue elasticity. Med Image Anal 2001;5:237–54.
47. Brown WE, Potter HG, Marx RG, et al. Magnetic resonance imaging appearance of cartilage repair in the knee. Clin Orthop Relat Res 2004;422:214–23.
48. Marlovits S, Singer P, Zeller P, et al. Magnetic resonance observation of cartilage repair tissue (MOCART) for the evaluation of autologous chondrocyte transplantation: determination of interobserver variability and correlation to clinical outcome after 2 years. Eur J Radiol 2006;57:16–23.
49. Welsch GH, Mamisch TC, Domayer SE, et al. Cartilage T2 assessment at 3-T MR imaging: in vivo differentiation of normal hyaline cartilage from reparative tissue after two cartilage repair procedures—initial experience. Radiology 2008;247: 153–61.
50. Gillis A, Bashir A, McKeon B, et al. Magnetic resonance imaging of relative glycosaminoglycan distribution in patients with autologous chondrocyte transplants. Invest Radiol 2001;36:743–8.
51. Mithoefer K, Williams RJ, Warren RF, et al. Prospective evaluation of the microfracture technique for treatment of articular cartilage lesions in the knee. J Bone Joint Surg 2005;87:1911–20.
52. Williams R III, Ranawat A, Carter T, et al. Fresh stored allografts for the treatment of osteochondral defects of the knee. J Bone Joint Surg 2007;89:718–26.
53. Sirlin CB, Brossmann J, Boutin RD, et al. Shell osteochondral allografts of the knee: comparison of MR imaging findings and immunologic responses. Radiology 2001; 219:35–43.

The Management of Sports-Related Concussion: Current Status and Future Trends

Mark Lovell, PhD

KEYWORDS

• Concussion • Sports management • Neurpsychology

The management of sports-related concussion is currently one of the most hotly debated issues in sports medicine, and there has been a sharp increase in research in this area over the past decade. Decisions regarding return to play following concussion represent one of the biggest challenges for the sports medicine practitioner. The team physician is often called on to make return-to-play decisions based on limited observation of the athlete and after a brief sideline evaluation. Furthermore, return-to-play decisions are often made under intense pressure against the backdrop of a noisy stadium/arena, where there is intense pressure to return the injured athlete to the playing field as quickly as possible. Therefore, the physician must balance the potential long-term effects of concussion against the short-term demands of the situation. This is no easy task.

As a result of concerns regarding both short-term and potential long-term sequelae of concussion, approximately 20 management guidelines have been published over the past 2 decades. However, these guidelines were largely based on the opinions of groups of experts rather than on systematic research.[1,2] Recent research has prompted a reevaluation and revision of prior guidelines, which has resulted in a corresponding revision in concussion management and return-to-play strategies. This article reviews new evidence-based trends in the evaluation and management of sports-related concussion and focuses specifically on practical suggestions for making return-to-play decisions.

DEFINITIONS OF CONCUSSION

Definitions of concussion have been evolving over the past 30 to 40 years and are likely to continue to evolve with ongoing discoveries in the neurosciences. Currently,

UPMC Sports Medicine Concussion Program, University of Pittsburgh Medical Center, Department of Orthopaedic Surgery, Pittsburgh, Pennsylvania 15228, USA
E-mail address: lovellmr@upmc.edu

Clin Sports Med 28 (2009) 95–111
doi:10.1016/j.csm.2008.08.008
0278-5919/08/$ – see front matter © 2008 Elsevier Inc. All rights reserved.

sportsmed.theclinics.com

there is no universally accepted definition of concussion. However, for the past 3 decades the definition originally proposed by the Committee on Head Injury Nomenclature of Neurologic Surgeons in 1966 has by far represented the most popular definition. This committee defined concussion as

"a clinical syndrome characterized by the immediate and transient posttraumatic impairment of neural function such as alteration of consciousness, disturbance of vision or equilibrium, etc., due to brain stem dysfunction."[3]

More recently, other definitions of concussion have been put forth. For example, in 1997, the American Academy of Neurology (AAN) defined concussion as

"Any trauma induced alteration in mental status that may or may not include a loss of consciousness."[4]

Authors of the AAN definition felt that the 1966 definition was too focused on brain stem dysfunction and loss of consciousness (LOC) and, therefore, did not consider the potential role of other brain structures (eg, cortical areas) and the potential importance of other markers of injury, such as confusion and amnesia.

PATHOPHYSIOLOGY OF CONCUSSION

Recent research regarding the subtle physiologic effects of concussion has lead to new insights into the pathophysiology of concussion. At the forefront of this area of research, Hovda and colleagues[5,6] described a metabolic dysfunction that occurs when cells immediately injured on concussive insult are exposed to dramatic changes in both their intracellular and extracellular environments. He suggested that these changes are the result of excitatory amino acid (EAA)-induced ionic shifts with increased Na/KATP-ase activation and resultant hyperglycolysis.[5] Thus, there is a high energy demand within the brain shortly after concussive injury. This process is accompanied by a decrease in cerebral blood flow, which is thought to cause widespread cerebral neurovascular constriction. The resulting "metabolic mismatch" between energy demand and energy supply within the brain has been postulated to result in cellular vulnerability. Hovda's research with rodents has suggested that this period of vulnerability can last up to 2 weeks.[6]

Hovda's initial research was groundbreaking and lead to an increased focus on the pathophysiology of this injury in human subjects. More recent research has examined the potential utility of functional magnetic resonance imaging (fMRI) as a viable tool for the assessment of neural processes following concussion. The technology is based on the measurement of specific correlates of brain activation, such as cerebral blood flow and oxygenation. In addition, fMRI involves no exposure to radiation and can be safely used in children. Furthermore, repeat evaluations can also be undertaken with minimal risk. This promotes the assessment of changes in neural substrata that may occur with mild concussion and makes it possible to track the injured athlete throughout the recovery process.

The Sports Medicine Concussion program at the University of Pittsburgh has recently completed a 5-year National Institute of Health funded study that has directly linked clinical recovery to resolution of abnormalities in cerebral blood flow in over 200 high school and collegiate athletes.[7] One of the major findings of this study was that athletes with abnormal fMRI studies within days of injury took twice as long to reach clinical recovery, compared with a group who did not initially show abnormalities on fMRI. **Figure 1** provides a graphic depiction of the fMRI of a 17-year-old female athlete who suffered a concussion without LOC. She struck the right temporal area of

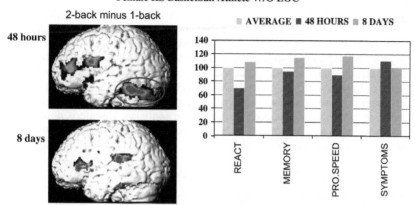

fMRI and NEUROPSYCHOLOGICAL TESTING
Female HS Basketball Athlete W/O LOC

Fig. 1. fMRI and imPACT case study data. fMRI and ImPACT data are presented for a 17-year-old female basketball player who suffered a concussion without LOC. At left, increased fMRI activation is shown within the cerebellum at 48 h post-injury, which resolves in a follow-up evaluation at 8 d posttrauma. At right, ImPACT deficits (relative to baseline) are noted at 48 h post-concussion in terms of reaction time, memory, and processing speed. The patient also reports an increase in symptoms. Resolution of ImPACT deficits are also evidenced at 8 d post-concussion.

her skull on a gymnasium floor while participating in a basketball game. She did not exhibit initial retrograde or anterograde amnesia but did exhibit a 30-second period of confusion. She also experienced dizziness and photosensitivity. The following morning, she complained of a right temporal headache and mild fatigue. She was referred to the University of Pittsburgh Medical Center (UPMC) Sports Concussion Program and was subsequently evaluated with both neuropsychological testing and an fMRI study. Her scan reveals an abnormal pattern of brain activation in posterior brain areas during the NBACK (number of stimuli back) memory task administered while she was in the scanner. This is thought to reflect an increase in brain area needed to complete the NBACK task following concussive injury.[7] The athlete was reevaluated 8 days post-injury. Her fMRI scan at this time period had normalized, as evidenced by activation of expected brain areas in the frontal and temporal lobes. Her neuropsychological test results (Immediate Post-Concussion Assessment and Cognitive Testing [ImPACT]) were congruent with this resolution of abnormal patterns visible through fMRI, demonstrating initial decline at 48 hours after injury and a return to pre-baseline levels at 8 days post-injury.

Although a promising tool, fMRI has yet to be widely implemented in clinical settings. At present, only a few laboratories are actively investigating the use of fMRI in sports-related head injury, although this is likely to change within the next few years.

At the current time, our understanding of the neurologic substrata of concussion is far from complete. However, existing research in both animal and human subjects raises important questions regarding the threat of increased vulnerability to injury following concussion in athletes. It has been postulated that metabolic dysfunction, until fully resolved, may lead to significantly increased neurologic vulnerability if a subsequent trauma (even minor) is sustained during the period of vulnerability. This metabolic dysfunction has been theoretically linked to second impact syndrome (SIS),[8] an often fatal syndrome that apparently occurs only in children and is the result of malignant brain swelling. It has also been suggested that changes in brain metabolism following concussion may be related to the less severe but more common post-concussion syndrome. Post-concussion syndrome occurs in approximately 10 to 20% of concussed athletes and refers to the experience of symptoms of concussion (eg, headache, fatigue, and memory impairment) that persist a month or more after injury. Although post-concussion syndrome can be evident after a single concussive event, it is felt that proper management of each concussive injury minimizes the potential for long-term or permanent post-concussive difficulties. Conversely, returning an athlete to participation before *complete* recovery may greatly increase the risk of lingering, long-term, or (rarely) even catastrophic neurologic sequelae. Therefore, acute assessment of concussion and determination of any existing signs/symptoms of injury prove critical to the safe management of the athlete.

ON-FIELD AND SIDELINE MANAGEMENT OF CONCUSSION

The diagnosis of cerebral concussion can be challenging under the best of circumstances. There may be no obvious direct trauma to the head and the concussed athlete is infrequently rendered unconscious. The athlete may also be unaware that he or she has been injured immediately after the injury and may not show any obvious signs of concussion, such as clumsiness, gross confusion, or obvious amnesia. To complicate this situation, athletes at all levels of competition may minimize or hide symptoms in an attempt to prevent their removal from the game, thus creating the potential for exacerbation of their injury.

INITIAL SIDELINE SIGNS AND SYMPTOMS OF EVALUATION AND RETURN TO PLAY

Table 1 provides a summary of common on-field signs and symptoms of concussion. It should be stressed that sideline presentation may vary widely form athlete to athlete, depending on the biomechanical forces involved, the athlete's prior history of injury, and numerous other factors. In reviewing the common signs and symptoms of concussion, it is important to stress that athletes vary greatly with regard to the symptoms they display following injury: Some athletes may present with primary cognitive difficulties (eg, concentration or memory difficulties), whereas others may suffer from headache, fatigue, or disruption of sleep. Therefore, a thorough assessment of *all* potential signs and symptoms of concussion symptoms should be conducted with every concussed athlete.

Headache is the most commonly reported symptom of injury and may be seen in up to 70% of athletes who sustain a concussion.[9] Although it is true that musculoskeletal headaches and other preexisting headache syndromes may complicate the assessment of post-concussion headache, any presentation of headache following a blow to the head or body should be managed conservatively. Most frequently, a concussion headache is described as a sensation of pressure in the skull that may be localized to one region of the head or may be generalized in nature. In some athletes (particularly athletes with a history of migraine), the headache may take the form of a vascular headache and may be unilateral and is often described as throbbing or pulsating. The headache may not develop immediately after injury and may develop in the minutes, or even hours, following injury. Therefore, it is essential to question the potentially concussed athlete regarding the development of symptoms beyond the first few minutes post-injury. It is also important to note that post-concussion headache is usually worsened with physical or cognitive exertion. Thus, if the athlete complains of worsening headache during workouts, post-concussion headache should be suspected, the athlete's activity level should be curtailed, and he or she should be closely monitored.

Table 1	
University of Pittsburgh signs and symptoms of concussion	
Signs Observed by Staff	**Symptoms Reported by Athlete**
Appears to be dazed or stunned	Headache
Is confused about assignment	Nausea
Forgets plays	Balance problems or dizziness
Is unsure of game, score, or opponent	Double or fuzzy/blurry vision
Moves clumsily	Sensitivity to light or noise
Answers questions slowly	Feeling sluggish or slowed down
Loses consciousness	Feeling "foggy" or groggy
Shows behavior or personality change	Concentration or memory problems
Forgets events before play (retrograde)	Change in sleep pattern (appears later)
Forgets events after hit (posttraumatic)	Feeling Fatigued

Although headache following a concussion does not necessarily constitute a medical emergency, a severe or progressively worsening headache, particularly when accompanied by vomiting or declining mental status, may signal a life-threatening situation and should prompt immediate transport to hospital and a CT scan of the brain.

Although headache is the most common symptom of concussion, concussion may occur without headache, and other signs or symptoms of injury should be carefully detailed and assessed. For example, athletes commonly experience blurred vision, changes in peripheral vision, or other visual disturbance (eg, seeing stars). These visual changes, in addition to photosensitivity and/or balance problems, are commonly associated with a blow to the back of the head (eg, head to turf). These athletes also often report increased fatigue, "feeling a step slow," or feeling sluggish. Fatigue is especially prominent in concussed athletes in the days following injury and is reported by a large number of athletes. In addition to these symptoms, cognitive or mental status changes are commonly seen immediately following injury. Athletes with any degree of mental status change should be managed conservatively.

ON-FIELD EVALUATION OF MENTAL STATUS AND MARKERS OF CONCUSSION

Appropriate management of the concussed athlete begins with an accurate assessment of the athlete on the field. As with any serious injury, the first priority is always to evaluate the athlete's level of consciousness and airway, breathing, and circulation (ABCs). The attending medical staff must always be prepared with an emergency action plan in the event the evacuation of a critically head- or neck-injured athlete is necessary. This plan should be familiar to all staff, be well delineated, and should be rehearsed in advance.

On ruling out more severe injury, acute evaluation continues with assessment of the concussion. First, the clinician should establish the presence of any LOC. By definition, LOC represents a state of brief coma in which the eyes are typically closed and the athlete is unresponsive to external stimuli. LOC is relatively rare and occurs in less than 10% of concussive injuries. Prolonged LOC (<1–2 minutes) in sports-related concussion is even less frequent[10] and athletes with LOC are typically unresponsive for only a few seconds. Obviously, any athlete with documented LOC should be managed conservatively and return to play is contraindicated. Occasionally, athletes demonstrate the "fencing reflex" on the field of play. The occurrence of fencing is characterized by the thrusting of the arms outward from the body and provides positive proof that LOC has occurred.

Confusion and amnesia are much more common than LOC following concussion. Confusion (ie, disorientation), by definition, represents impaired awareness and orientation to surroundings. Confusion is often manifested by the athlete appearing stunned, dazed, or glassy-eyed on the sideline. Confusion is frequently evident in athletes having difficulty with appropriate play calling, answering questions slowly or inappropriately, and/or repeating oneself during evaluation. Teammates are often the first to recognize that an athlete has been injured, given the difficulty in performing assignments on the field. On direct evaluation by the physician or athletic trainer, the athlete may be slow to respond. To properly assess the presence of confusion, the athlete can be asked simple orientation questions (eg, name, current stadium, city, opposing team, current month, and day).

A careful evaluation of amnesia is also of paramount importance in the acute evaluation of the concussed athlete because the duration of amnesia often provides important information regarding the severity of injury. Amnesia may be associated with loss of memory for events *preceding* or *following* injury. Posttraumatic amnesia refers to the period of amnesia *following* the injury until the athlete regains normal continuous memory functioning. As outlined in **Table 1**, on-field posttraumatic amnesia may be assessed through immediate and delayed (eg, 0, 5, and 15 minute) memory for 3 to 5 words (eg, girl, dog, green). The presence of posttraumatic amnesia, even for seconds, has been found to be highly predictive of post-injury neurocognitive deficits and persistent symptoms.[10]

Retrograde amnesia, although given less focus in the literature, may also be an important marker of concussion severity. Retrograde amnesia is defined as the inability to recall events occurring during the period *immediately preceding* trauma. To properly assess on-field retrograde amnesia, the athlete may be asked questions pertaining to details occurring just before the trauma that caused the concussion. As **Table 1** highlights, asking the athlete to recall details of the injury is a good starting point. From there, asking the athlete to recall the score of the game before the hit, events that occurred in the plays preceding the injury, and events that occurred in the first quarter/period or earlier in practice is a useful practical assessment strategy. It should be noted that the length of retrograde amnesia will typically "shrink" over time. For example, as recovery occurs, the length of retrograde amnesia may contract from hours to several minutes or even seconds. As is the case with posttraumatic amnesia, even seconds of retrograde amnesia may be considered to be potentially important with regard to prognosis for recovery.[11]

Several published studies have examined the relationship of on-field markers of concussion to outcome following concussion. Collins and colleagues[10] investigated the relationship between on-field markers of concussion severity and post-injury neurocognitive performance and symptom presentation in a group of 78 concussed high school and college athletes. Data from this study revealed that the presence of amnesia, not brief LOC, was most predictive of post-injury difficulties measured at 3 days post-injury. For example, athletes who had measurable post-concussive difficulties 3 days after injury (significant cognitive deficits and high degree of symptoms) were over *10 times more likely* to have exhibited *any* degree of retrograde amnesia following concussion when compared with athletes with good post-injury presentation (no cognitive deficits and no reported symptom). Similarly, athletes with poor performance were over 4 times more likely to have exhibited anterograde amnesia when evaluated on the field. It is important to note that LOC was *not* predictive of deficits following sports-related concussion. In another study that used computer-based testing, Erlanger and colleagues[11] found that athletes reporting memory problems following concussion had significantly more symptoms, longer duration of symptoms, and significant decreases on neurocognitive test performance. Data from these two studies directly contradicted prior grading systems of concussion that downplayed the predictive value of amnesia.

RETURN-TO-PLAY GUIDELINES: A BRIEF HISTORY AND REVIEW OF CURRENT TRENDS

Over the past 30 years, multiple concussion management guidelines have been published to provide guidance and direction for the sports-medicine practitioner in making complex return-to-play decisions.[1] The authors of each of these guidelines have also typically put forth corresponding "grading scales" designed to characterize the severity of the injury. Although these guidelines have no doubt resulted in improved care of the athlete, the existence of multiple guidelines also created significant confusion and sparked almost continuous debate. A detailed historical review of all past and current concussion guidelines is beyond the scope of this chapter; however, a brief review of 4 of the more recent and popular guidelines is provided in **Table 2**.

Cantu originally proposed his grading scale and management guidelines based on clinical experience.[12] However, Cantu was careful to emphasize that these guidelines were intended to supplement rather than replace clinical judgment. The original Cantu guidelines allowed return to play the day of injury if the athlete were symptom free both at rest and following physical exertion. For athletes who experienced any LOC (eg, Grade 3 concussion), a restriction of contact for 1 month was recommended. Athletes who had suffered a Grade 2 concussion were allowed to return to play in 2 weeks, if asymptomatic for a period of 7 days.

The Colorado Guidelines[13] were published in 1991 following the death of a high school athlete due to SIS and were published under the auspices of the Colorado Medical Society. These guidelines allowed same day return to play if symptoms cleared within 20 minutes of injury. For more severe injury (Grade 3 concussion), the AAN guideline recommended immediate transport to a hospital for further evaluation These guidelines were later revised under the sponsorship of the AAN (1997).[4] The AAN guidelines allowed return to competition the same day of injury if the athletes' signs and symptoms cleared within 15 minutes of injury. Grade 2 concussion was managed in a manner similar to the Colorado Guidelines, with return to competition within 1 week, if asymptomatic.

More recently, Cantu has amended his guidelines[14] to emphasize the duration of posttraumatic symptoms in grading the severity of the concussion and making return-to-play decisions. Grade 1 concussion was redefined by an absence of LOC and post-concussion signs or symptoms lasting less than 30 minutes. Same day return to competition was allowed only if the athlete was completely asymptomatic following the injury.

Although the above mentioned management guidelines reached their zenith of popularity during the 1980s and 1990s, in the late 1990s, sports medicine practitioners and their professional organizations began to question the scientific basis of these guidelines. This trend prompted the American Orthopaedic Society for Sports Medicine (AOSSM) to sponsor a workshop with the purpose of reevaluating current guidelines and establishing practical alternatives.[15] Although the AOSSM guidelines did not differ substantially from prior guidelines, this workshop started a trend away from the

Table 2
Recent concussion grading scales

Guideline	Grade 1	Grade 2	Grade 3
Cantu[6] (1986)	1. No LOC 2. Posttraumatic amnesia lasts less than 30 min	1. LOC lasts longer than 5 min OR 2. Posttraumatic amnesia lasts longer than 30 min	1. LOC lasts longer than 5 min OR 2. Posttraumatic amnesia lasts longer than 24 h
Colorado[22] (1991)	1. Confusion without amnesia 2. No LOC	1. Confusion with amnesia 2. No LOC	1. LOC (of any duration)
AAN[1] (1997)	1. Transient confusion 2. No LOC 3. Concussion symptoms or mental status changes resolve in less than 5 min	1. Transient confusion 2. No LOC 3. Concussion symptoms or mental status changes last longer than 15 min	1. LOC (brief or prolonged)
Cantu[7] (2001)	1. No LOC OR 2. Posttraumatic amnesia or signs/symptoms last longer than 30 min	1. LOC lasts less than 1 min OR 2. Posttraumatic amnesia lasts longer than 30 min but less than 24 h	1. LOC lasts more than 1 min OR 2. Posttraumatic amnesia lasts longer than 24 h OR 3. Post-concussion signs or symptoms last longer than 7 d

use of a numeric grading system for determination of return to play following concussion (eg, as developed by the Cantu, Colorado, and AAN guidelines). The AOSSM guidelines were also the first to stress more individualized management of injury, rather than applying general standards and protocols.

Yet another important evolutionary step with regard to concussion management took place in 2002 under the auspices of the Federation Internationale de Football Association (FIFA) in conjunction with the International Olympic Committee (IOC) and the International Ice Hockey Federation (IHF). The organizers of this meeting assembled a group of physicians, neuropsychologists, and sports administrators in Vienna, Austria, to continue to explore methods of reducing morbidity secondary to sports-related concussion. This group has subsequently been referred to at the Concussion in Sport (CIS) group. The deliberations that took place during this meeting lead to the publication of a document outlining recommendations for both the diagnosis and management of CIS.[16] One of the most important conclusions of this meeting was that none of the previously published concussion management guidelines were adequate to assure proper management of every concussion. The Vienna panel specifically emphasized the clinical utility of post-injury neuropsychological testing as a "cornerstone" of proper post-injury management and return-to-play decision making.

The recognition of neuropsychological testing as a key element of the post-concussion evaluation process represented a particularly important development in the diagnosis and management of the concussed athlete. The use of baseline neuropsychological testing was specifically recommended whenever possible, although there was an acknowledgment that neuropsychological testing was not available in many developing countries. In addition, a *graduated return-to-play* protocol was an important component of the CIS return-to-play protocol. The specific recommendations of the CIS group are presented in **Table 3**. It was specifically recommended that each step would, in most circumstances, be separated by 24 hours. Furthermore, it was recommended that any recurrence of concussive symptoms at a particular level of exertion should lead to the athlete dropping back to the previous level of exertion. In other words, if an athlete is asymptomatic at rest and develops a headache following light aerobic exercise, the athlete should return to complete rest. If the athlete developed headaches or other symptoms following heavy exertion, he/she should drop back to lighter exercise.

The CIS group published a second series of recommendations in 2005 [17] based on a meeting in Prague, the Czech Republic, in 2004. This paper reemphasized the need for individualized management of the athlete and continued to stress the need for neurocognitive assessment and graduated return to play following injury. In addition, the Prague conference suggested that concussions could be subdivided into "simple" (eg, resolving relatively quickly) and "complex" concussions (taking more than 10 days to recover). Unfortunately, however, no empiric support was put forth in support of this theoretic construct and it has yet to be validated.

MAKING DIFFICULT RETURN-TO-PLAY DECISIONS FOLLOWING CONCUSSION: IMPORTANT FACTORS

Once a concussed athlete has been removed from a game, the sports medicine physician is faced with the often challenging decision of when the athlete is safely able to return to play. Making return-to-play decisions, both on the field and during the post-injury management of injury (ie, days after injury), in athletes can be one of the most complex decisions facing the sports medicine physician. This represents a dynamic process that involves the evaluation of factors such as the severity of the injury (as measured by duration of LOC, amnesia, and confusion), the athlete's reported

---

Table 3
Vienna concussion conference: return-to-play recommendations. Athletes should complete the following stepwise process before return to play following concussion

1. Removal from contest following signs/symptoms of concussion.
2. No return to play in current game
3. Medical evaluation following injury
   a. Rule out more serious intracranial pathology
   b. Neuropsychological testing considered "cornerstone" of proper post-injury assessment pre-injury
4. Stepwise return to play
   a. No activity and rest until asymptomatic
   b. Light aerobic exercise
   c. Sport-specific training
   d. Noncontact drills
   e. Full-contact drills
   f. Game play

symptoms (eg, lingering headache, fatigue, photosensitivity, etc.), performance on neurocognitive testing, and the athlete's prior concussion history. With the more widespread use of neurocognitive testing, and the application of a more individualized management protocol, prospective data are now emerging that begin to shed light on individual factors that may play a role in the incidence, severity, and length of recovery regarding concussion. These factors are reviewed briefly in the next section.

Age and Developmental Level

Past concussion guidelines have assumed identical return-to-play criteria for athletes regardless of age. Based on these guidelines, it has traditionally been assumed that the speed of recovery is the same at all age groups and athletic levels. However, recent research has begun to expose potential differential age-related responses to concussive injury and has suggested the need for management protocols that are specific to different developmental levels.

A handful of published studies have directly examined recovery from concussion in college- versus high school aged athletes. Field and colleagues[18] measured both baseline and post-injury neuropsychological data in a sample of 53 athletes. Even though the college sample had a greater prior incidence of concussion, high school athletes were found to take longer to recover during an "in-study" concussion. This study suggested more protracted recovery from concussion in high school athletes. In a more recent study that used computer-based neuropsychological test results, Sim and colleagues[19] also found that high school students recovered more slowly than did college athletes.

Differences in cognitive performance have also been found between high school and professional football athletes, with high school athletes requiring considerably more time to recover.[20] Another recently published study[21] revealed the apparent heightened vulnerability to concussion in the younger athlete. Specifically, the issue of the "ding" or very mild concussion was examined in high school athletes aged 13 to 17 years.[21,22] One such study revealed that high school athletes with <15 minutes of on-field symptoms required at least 7 days before full neurocognitive and symptom recovery.[21] These findings suggest that all high school athletes diagnosed with concussion be removed from play during that contest.

As the above mentioned studies have suggested, there appears to be significant age-related differential response to concussive injury. It is also important to note that intangibles such as level of competition and overall risk/benefit analysis are also likely to be different at different levels (eg, pros versus amateur). Professional athletes may be willing to assume greater risk given obvious monetary and other considerations. Conversely, few parents would risk injury in a high school athlete who is unlikely to compete beyond high school.

Based on research conducted with more severe mild traumatic brain injury, several theories exist that might explain why younger athletes should be managed differently from older athletes. One such theory is that children may undergo more prolonged and diffuse cerebral swelling after traumatic brain injury, which suggests that they may be at an increased risk for secondary injury.[17] Furthermore; the immature brain may be up to 60 times more sensitive to glutamate,[23] a neurotransmitter involved in the metabolic cascade following concussion. These factors may lead to a longer recovery period and could increase the likelihood of permanent or severe neurologic deficit should re-injury occur during the recovery period. Such theory may help account for the finding that SIS has been found to occur only in child or adolescent athletes.[8]

History of Prior Concussion: Are the Effects of Concussion Cumulative?

In addition to the age of the athlete, the *concussion history* of the athlete may potentially be an important determinant of whether a concussed athlete can safely return to play. There is a growing body of evidence suggesting cumulative detrimental effects of multiple concussions. Cumulative effects of repeated head trauma have historically been associated with neurologic abnormalities documented in boxers.[24,25] However, more recently this topic has become an area of concern among other athletic populations. In a study of approximately 400 college football players, Collins and colleagues[26] found long-term subtle neurocognitive deficits in those suffering 2 or more concussions. Matser and colleagues[27] have also suggested that cumulative long-term consequences of repetitive blows to the head are often seen in professional soccer players. Even though data have been accumulating, there are no current reliable data available to determine *how many* concussions should preclude return to participation or force retirement from sport. A series of papers have recently been published using data gathered in professional football players. In a study that evaluated a sample of National Football League (NFL) athletes, Pellman and colleagues[28] found that athletes who had a history of 3 or more concussions demonstrated a similar pattern of signs and symptoms compared with those who had experienced a single injury. In an additional study of NFL athletes, Pellman and colleagues[29] did not find poorer neuropsychological test performance in a group with multiple injuries compared with a group without multiple injuries. A recent study that surveyed a sample of retired NFL athletes suggested that retired athletes who reported 3 or more concussions were more likely to report symptoms of depression as well as cognitive impairment. However, it must be emphasized that this study relied solely on the self-report of the retired athletes and their retrospective recall of past injuries.[30] A large-scale study is currently being conducted under the auspices of the NFL Committee on Mild Traumatic Brain Injury, which is hoped to better address this issue. Specifically, this study will subject a large sample of retired NFL athletes to comprehensive brain imaging, neuropsychological testing, and a formal neurologic evaluation. It is hoped that this study will help to answer some of the remaining questions regarding the relative importance of multiple concussions.

Are there Sex Differences in Recovery from Concussion?

As noted throughout this chapter, the management of sports-related concussion has been an evolving process. With our increasing understanding of the underlying pathophysiology of concussion has come a more refined understanding of important factors that may influence who sustains a concussion and how quickly they recover from injury. Very recently, new evidence has surfaced to suggest that there may be gender differences with regard to concussion. Large-scale epidemiologic data collected through the High School Reporting Information Hotline (RIO) and the National Collegiate Athletic Association (NCAA) have reported that females have a higher rate of concussion in comparison with their male counterparts.[31] Furthermore, neuropsychological evidence has indicated that females are cognitively impaired 1.7 times more frequently than males.[32] Most recently, the authors' laboratory at the University of Pittsburgh has compared a large sample of male and female soccer players, adjusting for body mass index, and found that females had significantly more post-concussive symptoms as well as poorer performance on a computer-based test that measured memory, processing speed, and reaction time (ImPACT).[33] What remains unclear at this point in time is the potential reason for these gender differences. While the difference in neck strength between males and females has been suggested,[34] it is also possible that there are gender-specific differences in brain physiology that may be contributing to these findings. It is hoped that continued research in this area will clarify the complex factors that might be involved.

THE ROLE OF NEUROPSYCHOLOGICAL TESTING IN MAKING RETURN-TO-PLAY DECISIONS

The development of neuropsychological testing as a diagnostic tool in sports medicine is a relatively recent development that initially took place in the mid 1980s within the context of a large multisite research project undertaken by Barth and his colleagues[35] at the University of Virginia. This study demonstrated the potential utility of neuropsychological test procedures to document cognitive recovery within the first week following concussion. However, this study did not result in the widespread adoption of neuropsychological testing in organized athletics at the clinical level. In the early 1990s, a series of events transpired that shifted the use of neuropsychological testing in sports to the clinical arena. First, injuries to a number of high-profile professional athletes resulted in the implementation of baseline neuropsychological testing by a number of NFL teams in the mid 1990s.[36] Similarly, following career-ending injuries in the National Hockey League (NHL), the NHL mandated baseline neuropsychological testing for all athletes.[37] In addition to the increased use of neuropsychological testing in professional sports, several large-scale studies of collegiate athletes were undertaken. These studies further verified that neuropsychological testing yielded useful clinical information.[26,38] Specifically, neuropsychological testing allowed a baseline/post-injury analysis of the subtle aspects of cognitive function likely affected by concussive injury, thus providing objective data to make more informed decisions regarding return to play.

The use of traditional neuropsychological testing (eg, paper and pencil testing) resulted in the rapid expansion of our knowledge regarding concussions and became a popular clinical tool within the professional ranks. However, the more widespread application of testing within the college ranks has been limited due to practical and economic constraints. Furthermore, neuropsychological testing at the high school level was extremely limited before the year 2003. This fact is disturbing given that the vast majority of at-risk athletes fall within the high school ranks and below. Traditional neuropsychological testing has proven to be too time consuming and costly for many amateur organizations, and the expansion of testing has also been limited by a shortage of trained neuropsychologists to oversee the administration and interpretation of the assessment process. As a result of these inherent limitations of traditional assessment and in parallel with the widespread proliferation of the microcomputer, several researchers have begun to develop computer-based neuropsychological testing procedures.

Computer-based neuropsychological testing procedures have a number of advantages and relatively few disadvantages when compared with traditional neuropsychological testing procedures. First, the use of computers allows the evaluation of large numbers of student athletes with minimal manpower. For example, through the program at the University of Pittsburgh, up to 20 athletes were routinely evaluated simultaneously in a high school or college computer laboratory. This promotes the assessment of an entire football team within a reasonable time period using minimal human resources. Second, data acquired through testing can be easily stored in a specific computer or computer network and can, therefore, be accessed at a later date (eg, following injury). Not only does this promote the efficient clinical evaluation of the athlete but also greatly expands the possibilities for research. Third, the use of the microcomputer promotes the more accurate measurement of cognitive processes such as reaction time and information processing speed. In fact, computerized assessment allows for the evaluation of response times that are accurate to the 1/100 of a second, whereas traditional testing allows for accuracy only to 1 to 2 seconds. This increased accuracy will no doubt increase the *validity* of test results in detecting subtle changes in neurocognitive processes. Fourth, the use of the computer allows for the randomization of test stimuli, which should help to improve *reliability* across multiple administration periods, minimizing the "practice effects" that naturally occur with multiple exposures to the stimuli. These practice effects have clouded the interpretation of research studies and have also presented an obstacle for the clinician evaluating the true degree of neurocognitive deficit following injury. Limiting the influence of practice effects on testing allows a direct interpretation of post-injury data to the athlete's baseline to determine whether full cognitive recovery has occurred. Finally, computer-based approaches allow for the rapid dissemination of clinical information into a coherent clinical report that can be easily interpreted by the sports medicine clinician. In summary, there are many benefits derived from a computer-based approach insofar as the technology has appropriate sensitivity, reliability, and validity in measuring the subtle aspects of concussive injury.

CURRENT APPROACHES TO COMPUTER-BASED NEUROPSYCHOLOGICAL TESTING

At the current time, there are several computer-based management approaches under development. All of these test batteries are structured to help provide the sports medicine practitioner with neurocognitive data to better determine return to play and other management issues following concussive injury. Specifically, 4 computer-based models have been reviewed in the scientific literature. These include ImPACT Cog-State, Headminders-CRI, and Automated Neuropsychological Assessment Metric (ANAM). Differences do exist between these test batteries and each is at different stages of validation. Clearly, issues such as *sensitivity*, *reliability*, and *validity* of the respective test batteries should be given careful scrutiny before implementation is adopted. In addition, issues regarding test selection, cognitive domains measured, details of the clinical report, and consultation options for each instrument should be carefully reviewed before implementation. A detailed review of these critical issues for each computerized battery is beyond the scope of this article. The reader is urged, however, to adequately explore the advantages and disadvantages of each test battery before incorporating a particular test battery into their injury management system. Again, it is imperative that clinicians understand that the cognitive data derived from these instruments are not a panacea to concussion management. Rather, these tools provide "one piece of the puzzle" and should be used only as a component of the overall medical evaluation.

Computerized neuropsychological testing is beginning to create heated interest within the sports medicine arena. The ability to collect objective, sensitive, and detailed neurobehavioral information pertaining to the athlete's post-concussive status is of obvious merit and is rapidly becoming the standard of care in sports medicine. For example, such an approach to injury is systematic and individually tailored, rather than applying general standards (eg, grading systems) to concussion management that lack empiric validation. In addition, computer-based neuropsychological assessment has been demonstrated to have predictive value above and beyond reliance on athlete self-report alone. For example, van Kampen and colleagues[39] documented that the use of neuropsychological testing in addition to self-reported symptoms resulted in greatly enhanced identification of concussed athletes compared with reliance on symptoms alone.

Other Diagnostic Tools

As noted previously, the diagnosis and management of concussion should involve multiple assessment modalities. Although athletes often present with cognitive difficulties that can be detected by neuropsychological testing, some athletes demonstrate noncognitive signs or symptoms. Balance dysfunction following concussion is relatively common, occurring in up to 40% of concussed athletes.[40] Therefore, it is very useful to evaluate balance both immediately after injury and throughout the recovery process. Disruption of balance can be secondary to trauma to the brain or may also be the result of trauma to the vestibular system. At a minimum, an assessment of balance should involve an analysis of postural sway (eg, athlete standing with feet together with eyes closed). Riemann and colleagues[41] have used a more comprehensive yet portable evaluation of balance (the Balance Error Scoring System or BESS). This evaluation involves the athlete performing a series of balance exercises while standing on a piece of foam with eyes closed. The BESS represents a practical and useful balance assessment test that should be used to augment the return-to-play decision-making process.

One relatively new development in the evaluation of concussion is the use of sophisticated visual tracking technology. Slobounov and his colleagues[42] have found balance deficits that were induced by visual field motion that lasted up to 30 days in a sample of brain-injured athletes. This line of research may yield clinically useful information in the near future.

A RETURN-TO-PLAY PROTOCOL FOLLOWING CONCUSSION

Based on recent research regarding recovery from concussion and the Vienna international consensus statement,[16] the UPMC return-to-play protocol involves the graduated return to play of the athlete to competition based on his or her progression through several steps in the recovery process. First and foremost, it is strongly felt that athletes who have either abnormal neuropsychological testing results or are symptomatic should not be returned to play following injury until they are asymptomatic and any cognitive difficulties have resolved.

As reviewed earlier in the chapter, it is also strongly suggested that younger athletes (eg, high school age and below) should not be returned to play during the game in which they were injured. This allows for closer evaluation of evolving signs and symptoms and will help to prevent more severe injury. Formal neuropsychological testing the day after injury is recommended to assess initial neurocognitive status. It is also important to reevaluate the athlete regularly with regard to reported at-rest symptoms.

Once the athlete is symptom-free at rest, graduated aerobic exertional testing is suggested to check for the return of symptoms such as headache, dizziness, nausea, or mental fogginess. When the athlete becomes asymptomatic following exertion, neuropsychological testing should also be completed and the athlete's test results should be compared with the baseline. If pre-injury baseline neuropsychological testing has not been previously completed, the athlete's test performance should be compared with normative standards for his or her age and gender. Finally, it should be emphasized that this protocol is based on research with younger, primarily high school aged subjects and the management of the older athlete (eg, college or professional) may vary. It is hoped that recent large-scale research projects within the NFL and NHL will shed additional light on the management of concussion in professional athletes.

CONCLUSIONS AND FUTURE DIRECTIONS

This article has focused on new developments in the management of sports-related concussion. Specifically, it has been emphasized that the clinical management of concussion is evolving rapidly and there is still much to learn about both the short- and long-term consequences of injury. As increasingly more research studies are designed to investigate the biomechanics, pathophysiology, and clinical course of sports-related concussion, our management strategies will continue to evolve over the next 5 to 10 years. Although standards for concussion management continue to change in response to new and increasingly sophisticated research, one trend has become particularly clear over the past 10 years: Concussion management has become increasingly individualized. This trend is likely to continue. The 1980s and 1990s were characterized by the publication of multiple concussion "guidelines," which made specific return-to-play recommendations based on duration of concussion markers, such as LOC, amnesia, and so forth. However, there has been recent acknowledgment by leaders in the field that guidelines may have limited utility, and the focus has shifted to a more individualized approach based on the establishment of an absence of any clinical symptomatology and establishment of normal brain function before return to play.[2] The diagnostic techniques outlined in this article will probably play an important role in the clinical management of concussion.

REFERENCES

1. Collins MW, Lovell MR, McKeag DB. Current issues in managing sports concussion. JAMA 1999;282:2283–5.
2. Grindel SH, Lovell MR, Collins MW. The assessment of sports-related concussions: the evidence behind neuropsychological testing and management. Clin J Sport Med 2001;11:134–43.
3. Congress of Neurological Surgeons. Committee on head injury nomenclature: glossary of head injury. Clin Neurosurg 1966;12:386–94.
4. American Academy of Neurology. Practice parameter: the management of concussion in sports (summary statement). Report of the quality standards subcommittee. Neurol 1997;48:581–5.
5. Bergschneider M, Hovda DA, Shalmon E. Cerebral hyperglycolysis following severe human traumatic brain injury: a positron emission tomography study. J Neurosurg 2003;86:241–51.
6. Hovda DA, Prins M, Becker DP. Neurobiology of concussion. In: Bailes JE, Lovell MR, Maroon JC, editors. Sports Related Concussion. St. Louis (MO): Quality Medical Publishing; 1999. p. 12–51.
7. Lovell MR, Pardini JE, Welling J, et al. Functional brain abnormalities are related to clinical recovery and time to return to play in athletes. Neurosurgery 2007; 61(2):352–9.
8. Cantu R, Voy R. Second impact syndrome: a risk in any sport. Phys Sports Med 1995;23:27–36.
9. Collins MW, Field M, Lovell MR, et al. Relationship between post-concussion headache and neuropsychological test performance in high school athletes. Am J Sports Med 2003;31:168–73.
10. Collins MW, Iverson GL, Lovell MR, et al. On-field predictors of neuropsychological and symptom deficit following sports-related concussion. Clin J Sport Med 2003;13:222–9.
11. Erlanger D, Kausik, Cantu R, Barth JT, et al. Symptom-based assessment of the severity of concussion. J Neurosurg 2003;98:34–9.

12. Cantu RC. Cerebral concussion in sport: management and prevention. Phys Sports Med 1992;14:64–74.
13. Kelly JP, Nichols JS, Filley CM. Concussion in sports: guidelines for the prevention of catastrophic outcome. JAMA 1991;266:2867–9.
14. Cantu RC. Posttraumatic retrograde and anterograde amnesia: pathophysiology and implications in grading and safe return to play. J Athl Train 2001;36:244–8.
15. Wojyts ED, Hovda D, Landry G, et al. Concussion in sports. Am J Sports Med 1999;27:676–86.
16. Aubry M, Cantu R, Dvorak J, et al. Summary of the first international conference on concussion in sport. Clin J Sport Med 2002;12:6–11.
17. McCrory P, Johnston K, Meeuwisse W, et al. Summary of the second international conference on concussion in sport. Br J Sports Med 2005;39(4):196–204.
18. Field M, Collins MW, Lovell MR, et al. Does age play a role in recovery from sports related concussion? A comparison of high school and collegiate athletes. J Pediatr 2003;142:546–53.
19. Sim A, Terryberry-Spohr L, Wilson KR. Prolonged recovery of memory functioning after mild traumatic brain injury in adolescent athletes. J Neurosurg 2008;108(3):511–6.
20. Pellman E, Lovell MR, Viano DC, et al. Concussion in professional football: recovery of NFL and high school athletes assessed by computerized testing-Part 12. Neurosurgery 2006;58(2):263–4.
21. Lovell MR, Collins MW, Iverson GL, et al. Recovery from mild concussion in high school athletes. J Neurosurg 2003;98:296–301.
22. Lovell MR, Collins MW, Iverson GL, et al. Grade 1 or "ding" concussions in high school athletes. Am J Sports Med 2004;32(1):460–7.
23. Pickles W. Acute general edema of the brain in children with head injuries. N Engl J Med 1950;242:607–11.
24. Jordan BD, Relkin NR, Ravdin LD. Apolipoprotein E e4 associated with chronic traumatic brain injury in boxing. JAMA 1997;278:136–40.
25. Roberts GW, Allsop B, Bruton C. The occult aftermath of boxing. J Neurol Neurosurg Psychiatr 1990;53:373–8.
26. Collins MW, Grindel SH, Lovell MR, et al. DM Relationship between concussion and neuropsychological performance in college football players. JAMA 1999;282:964–70.
27. Matser E, Kessels A, Lezak M. Neuropsychological impairment in amateur soccer players. JAMA 1999;282:971–4.
28. Pellman EJ, Viano DC, Casson IR, Tucker AM, et al. Concussion in professional football: repeat injuries-part 4. Neurosurg 2004;55(4):873–6.
29. Pellman EJ, Lovell MR, Viano DC, et al. Concussion in professional football: neuropsychological testing-part 6. Neurosurg 2004;55(6):1303–5.
30. Guskiewicz KM, Marshall SW, Bailes J, et al. Association between recurrent concussion and late-life cognitive impairment in retired professional football players. Neurosurg 2005;57(4):719–26.
31. Gessel LM, Fields SK, Collins CL, et al. Concussions among United States high school and collegiate athletes. J Athl Train 2007;42(4):495–503.
32. Brosheck DK, Kaushik T, Freeman JR, et al. Sex differences in outcome following sports-related concussion. J Neurosurg 2005;102(5):856–63.
33. Colvin A, Mullen, J, Lovell MR, et al. The effects of gender and concussion history on recovery in soccer athletes. Paper presented at the American orthopaedic society for Sports Medicine, Orlando (FLA), 2008.

34. Tierney RT, Sitler MR, Swanik CB, et al. Gender differences in head-neck segment dynamic stabilization during head acceleration. Med Sci Sports Exerc 2005;37(2):272–9.

35. Barth JT, Alves WM, Ryan TV, et al. Mild head injury in sports. In: Levin HS, Eisenberg H, Benton A, editors. Mild head injury. Oxford: Oxford University Press; 1989. p. 257–75.

36. Lovell MR. Evaluation of the professional athlete. In: Bailes JE, Lovell MR, Maroon JC, editors. Sports-related concussion. St. Louis (MO): Quality Medical Publishing, Inc.; 1999. p. 200–14.

37. Lovell MR, Burke CJ. Concussion management in professional hockey. In: Cantu RE, editor. Neurologic athletic head and spine injury. Philadelphia: WB Saunders; 2000.

38. Echemendia RJ, Putukian M, Macklin. Neuropsychological test performance prior to and following sports-related mild traumatic brain injury. Clin J Sport Med 2001; 11:23–31.

39. van Kampen DA, Lovell MR, Pardini JE, et al. The "value added" of neurocognitive testing after sports-related concussion. Am J Sports Med 2006;34(10): 1630–5.

40. Collins MW, Lovell MR, Iverson GL, et al. Cumulative effects of sports concussion in high school athletes. Neurosurg 2002;51:1175–81.

41. Riemann BL, Guskiewicz KM. Effects of mild head injury on postural stability as measured through clinical balance testing. J Athl Train 2000;35(1):19–25.

42. Slobounov S, Tutwiler R, Sabastianelli W, et al. Alteration of postural responses to visual field motion in mild traumatic brain injury. Foundations of Sports-Related Brain Injury 2006;59(1):134–9.

Treatment of Tendon and Muscle Using Platelet-Rich Plasma

Allan Mishra, MD[a],*, James Woodall, Jr., MD[b], Amy Vieira, PA-C[a]

KEYWORDS

- Platelet-rich plasma • PRP • Growth factors • Tendon
- Muscle • Tendonitis

Musculoskeletal injuries and impairments result in over 100 million office visits in the United States per year. Tendons and muscle-related issues account for a significant percentage of these visits. As our population ages and remains active, the number of orthopedic-related problems will rise dramatically.[1] Younger and older patients expect faster recovery from their injuries with less invasive procedures. Within this landscape, PRP has become a potential standalone or adjunctive treatment.

The concept of using the growth factors within PRP to help heal wounds dates back to the early 1980s.[2] Its use in orthopedic surgery, however, began during this decade and initially focused on the augmentation of bone grafting. The efficacy of PRP to accelerate bone healing continues to be debated in the literature.[3–8] Employing PRP to augment tendon healing, however, has been advocated only recently.[9,10]

PLATELET-RICH PLASMA BIOCHEMISTRY

PRP is a bioactive component of whole blood. The specific elements of PRP have not been uniformly defined in the literature. PRP, in general, has a higher concentration of platelets compared with baseline blood. Clinically valuable PRP, however, typically contains 1 million platelets or more per microliter.[11] Some authors define PRP as only platelets whereas others note that PRP may also have increased concentrations of white blood cells. The white blood cells within some forms of PRP contain important cytokines and enzymes. For example, Horsburgh and colleagues[12] found that platelet-derived mediators may be responsible for increased monocyte adherence in vitro. This adherence may be important for long-term tissue regeneration that is macrophage

Financial Disclosure: Allan Mishra has a license agreement with Biomet Biologics.
[a] Department of Orthopedic Surgery, Menlo Medical Clinic, Stanford University Medical Center, 1300 Crane Street, Menlo Park, CA 94025, USA
[b] Department of Orthopedic Surgery, University of Mississippi Medical Center, 2500 North State Street, Jackson, MS 39216, USA
* Corresponding author. 340 August Circle, Menlo Park, CA 94025.
E-mail address: am@totaltendon.com (A. Mishra).

Clin Sports Med 28 (2009) 113–125
doi:10.1016/j.csm.2008.08.007
0278-5919/08/$ – see front matter

mediated. Importantly, in vitro studies have also found that PRP significantly inhibits the growth of *Staphylococcus aureus* and *Escherichia coli*. In one of these studies, PRP was found to have no activity against *Pseudomonas aeruginosa*, *Klebsiella pneumoniae*, or *Enterococcus faecalis*.[13,14]

PRP activation and the pH of PRP are other parameters that are being debated in the literature. Thrombin and calcium have historically been used to activate platelets. This combination results in the formation of a gel that may be used in open surgery but cannot be injected even through a large-gauge needle. Thrombin and calcium activation results in rapid release of contents of the granules within platelets. This requires immediate use of the PRP. Platelets, however, can be slowly activated by exposure to tendon-derived collagen.[15] This can produce in vivo activation and allows for administration of PRP through a small-gauge needle. Variations in partial activation with calcium are also being explored.[16] Liu and colleagues[17] have also found the release of growth factors from PRP to be pH dependent.

When platelets are activated either ex vivo or in vivo, they release the growth factors and proteins that reside within their alpha and dense granules. The alpha granules contain cytokines including platelet-derived growth factor, transforming growth factor-β, and vascular endothelial growth factor, among many others (**Table 1**).[18] Concentrations of these growth factors rise linearly with increasing platelet concentration.[11,19] After release, the cytokines are free to bind to transmembrane receptors on the surface of local or circulating cells. They then initiate intracellular signaling, which results in the expression of proteins responsible for cellular chemotaxis, matrix synthesis, and proliferation. Tissue regeneration through angiogenesis, extracellular matrix production, and collagen synthesis is orchestrated by the autocrine and paracrine effects of the growth factors. Everts and colleagues[20] have elegantly outlined the electron micrographic properties of how PRP releases these proteins. Properly prepared PRP in an unactivated form clearly reveals an abundance of platelets in a photomicrograph at high power (**Fig. 1**).[21]

Much emphasis has been placed on alpha granules but dense granules also play a role in tissue modulation and regeneration. The dense granules contain adenosine, serotonin, histamine, and calcium.

Adenosine is a nucleoside that plays an important role in many biochemical processes, including transfer of energy. Adenosine is a primary cytoprotective agent that prevents tissue damage. Adenosine receptor activation has been shown to have an anti-inflammatory effect during the inflammatory process associated with diabetic nephropathy.[23] In laboratory studies, adenosine A2A receptor agonists applied topically to diabetic foot wounds have been effective in tissue repair and reconstruction and their effect on difficult wounds in humans is currently under investigation.[24] Adenosine also has the ability to increase IL-10 production by macrophages in some cases.[25] This increase in IL-10 could indicate a change in the character of the

Table 1		
Selected growth factors within platelet-rich plasma[19,22]		
Growth Factor	**Actions**	
Platelet-derived growth factor	Chemoattractive for mesenchymal stem cells and monocytes	
Transforming growth factor- β	Mitogen for fibroblasts and enhances extracellular matrix production	
Vascular endothelial growth factor	Stimulates angiogenesis	

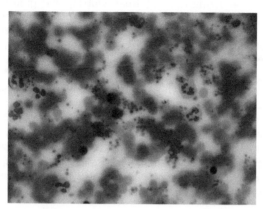

Fig. 1. Photomicrograph of PRP. Note high concentration of platelets.

macrophage to an anti-inflammatory state. In other instances, it appears that adenosine can function to activate macrophages to produce pro-inflammatory cytokines, IL-1 and IL-18.[26]

Serotonin is a monoamine neurotransmitter. This hormone can be exponentially more effective at increasing capillary permeability than even histamine.[27] Serotonin also acts as a chemoattractant for fibroblasts and increases their proliferation. Interestingly, macrophage cells have receptors that are sensitive to serotonin. Serotonin injected locally into tissue induces an influx of macrophages into that tissue.[28] Serotonin has also been shown to effect macrophages by suppression of IFN–gamma-induced 1a expression at sites of inflammation.[29] These data suggest strong interactions between serotonin and macrophages. This relationship and the particular effect serotonin has on cellular interactions should be considered when evaluating the effects of PRP on inflammation and healing.

Histamine is a biogenic amine involved in local immune responses. Locally, it also acts as a vasodilator. Histamine enhances permeability of the microvascular system of capillaries and venules. This increased permeability is due to the contraction of endothelial cells and removal of fenestrated diaphragms blocking gaps in the endothelial lining.[30] At the time of injury, histamine is released, acting as a vasodilator that actively increases endothelial membrane permeability. This increase in membrane permeability allows inflammatory and immune cells greater access to marginate and enter the local area. Histamine is also a strong activator of macrophages.

Calcium is the final component of the dense granules. Involvement of calcium in wound healing is mainly in keratinocyte proliferation and differentiation. Skin fibroblasts require calcium but are far less sensitive than keratinocytes to its effects. Calcium may also be required in epidermal cell migration and regeneration in the remodeling phase. Although calcium dressings are meant to serve in the hemostatic phase of healing, it is unclear whether their effect carries over into the later remodeling phase. The effect of calcium is essential in wound management, and the calcium content within the dense granules of platelets may play a vital role in its delivery to the site of injury.[31]

The unique combination and concentration of bioactive molecules that exist within PRP have profound effects on the inflammatory, proliferative, and remodeling phases of wound healing. Researchers worldwide are evaluating how PRP produces these effects. Not all cytokines within PRP have been characterized. These cytokines also exist in hyperphysiologic concentrations in PRP when compared with whole blood.

Since healing of tendon and muscle is similar to wound healing in some respects, PRP has great potential to improve soft tissue healing. The concept of using PRP to restore tendons and muscle after injuries is explored in this context.

TENDON INJURIES AND HEALING

Tendon injuries and disorders come in many forms (**Table 2**). The generic term, tendinopathy, is best used to describe these many forms. The spectrum of problems ranges from acute tendonitis to chronic tendinosis to full-thickness tearing. Extrinsic factors, for example, a hooked acromion in the shoulder, combined with intrinsic factors, such as age-related degeneration, can contribute to tendinopathy. Repetitive microtrauma or exposure to fluoroquinolone antibiotics has also been implicated.[32,33] Genetic factors, matrix metalloproteases (MMPs), and apoptosis may further contribute to tendon degeneration.[34]

Tendon healing occurs through 3 phases: inflammation, proliferation, and remodeling. These overlapping phases are controlled by a variety of growth factors. They are also linked through complex cellular signaling cascades.[22,36] For example, the temporal expression of growth factors has been reported to be important in supraspinatus tendon healing.[37] Since PRP contains many of these cytokines and cells in hyperphysiologic doses, it may be a reasonable choice to help initiate or accelerate tendon healing. The use of PRP for tendon disorders is presently being investigated for significant tendon disorders, such as chronic severe tendinosis, or in combination with surgery for complete tendon tears.

Use of PRP in Tendinopathy

In vitro studies have found that PRP can enhance human stromal and mesenchymal stem cell proliferation.[38] Conversely, Woodall and colleagues[39,40] found that PRP suppresses macrophage proliferation and IL-1 production within the first 72 hours after exposure. This differential induction of cells has important implications for tendon and muscle healing. It may be possible for PRP to initially inhibit excess inflammation while stimulating proliferation and maturation. This may be especially important in preventing the fibrous scar tissue healing that occurs with macrophage-mediated tendon-to-bone healing.[41] Future studies should evaluate the possibility that PRP may also stimulate tendon stem cells that have recently been identified.[42]

Equine and human cell culture studies support the use of PRP for the treatment of tendon injuries and disorders. Schnabel and colleagues[43] reported enhanced type I

Table 2 Types of tendon problems	
Type of Tendon Problem[35,36]	Findings
True tendonitis	Associated with acute increase in activity, eg, patellar tendonitis with hill running
Tendinosis	Common, misdiagnosed as "tendonitis." A chronic degeneration of a tendon, eg, "tennis elbow"
Torn tendon	Common, can occur with trauma or spontaneously through chronic tendinosis, eg, Achilles tear or rotator cuff tear
Tendinopathy	Generic term for tendon disorder
Tendon-related pain	What the patient complains of and what the clinician needs to treat

collagen gene expression in PRP-cultured tendon cells, with no concomitant increase in catabolic molecules, such as matrix metalloproteinase 3 (MMP-3). Other authors, however, have found that PRP not only stimulates human tenocyte proliferation and total collagen production but also slightly increases MMP-3 expression.[44] Anitua and colleagues[45] reported that the balance between TGF-β and other secreted cytokines may control angiogenesis and fibrosis.

Aspenberg and Virchenko reported greater maturation in tendon callus when PRP was used to augment rat Achilles tendon tears. They also reported increased force to failure and ultimate stress in PRP-treated animals.[46,47] In a landmark study, Kajikawa and colleagues[48] found that PRP enhances the mobilization of circulation-derived cells to an area of injection. They also found that PRP induced type I collagen production and increased the proliferation of macrophages at 3 and 7 days. This article did not, however, measure macrophage proliferation in the first 48 hours, so it is not possible to directly compare it to the work of Woodall et al, which showed initial macrophage suppression during that period.

Mishra and Pavelko were the first to report the use of PRP for patients considering surgery for chronic severe elbow tendinosis (**Fig. 2**).[9] All of the patients had failed a standardized nonoperative treatment protocol. In this prospective, controlled pilot study using unactivated and buffered PRP, the authors found 60% improvement in pain scores for PRP-treated patients versus a 16% improvement in control patients 8 weeks after treatment. This was a small, nonrandomized study. At final follow-up (mean, 25.6 months; range, 12–38 months), however, the PRP patients reported over 90% reduction in pain compared with pre-treatment scores. Ninety-three percent of patients were also fully satisfied with the treatment. A double-blind prospective randomized trial of 230 patients using this protocol in the United States has been initiated. No significant complications or worsening of symptoms has been reported using this technique.

Anitua and colleagues[45] found faster recovery in athletes undergoing PRP-enhanced Achilles tendon repair. In their study, athletes treated with surgery and PRP were compared with a retrospective control group of athletes treated with surgery alone. The PRP patients recovered range of motion earlier, had no wound complications, and returned to training activities in less time than control patients. The cross-sectional area of the PRP-treated tendons was also smaller than that in nontreated tendons when measured by ultrasound. Randelli and colleagues[49] recently

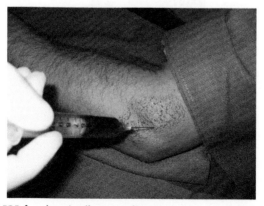

Fig. 2. Injection of PRP for chronic elbow tendinosis.

reported a case series of patients treated with PRP-augmented arthroscopic rotator cuff repairs. They found the technique to be safe without any reported complications and all patients recovered full passive range of motion within 1 month post-treatment. Gamradt and colleagues[50] reported on another technique for potentially enhancing rotator cuff repair with a different form of PRP. This method is presently being evaluated in a prospective, randomized trial.

Several other trials are underway in the United States and Europe to clarify the value of PRP for tendon injuries. Gosen and colleagues[51] are using unactivated PRP in a prospective double-blind randomized controlled trial of 100 patients to test PRP against cortisone in patients with chronic lateral epicondylar tendinosis. Preliminary data from their study find PRP patients demonstrating more reduction in pain and higher DASH scores at 24 weeks. Aspenberg and colleagues are presently conducting a prospective, randomized trial of PRP-augmented Achilles tendon repairs in humans. They will also be able to report biomechanical data because they are implanting tantulum balls above and below the repair site. This will allow measurement of tendon elongation postoperatively. Similar findings in the United States and Europe also support the use of PRP in the treatment of chronic Achilles tendinopathy (**Figs. 3** and **4**). (Mishra, personal communication, June 2008).

The Role of PRP in Muscle Injuries

Muscle injuries may be caused by a contusion by way of a direct blow, a strain, or occasionally a laceration. Rapid eccentric contraction is responsible for many of these injuries and the musculotendinous junction is the most common location of injury. Contact, sprinting, and jumping sports yield the most muscle injuries.[52] Although imaging studies may be included in the workup, diagnosis is based largely on patient history and physical examination. While there is no universal classification system for muscle injuries, the most common one has been adapted from Ryan's system (**Table 3**).[53]

Muscle healing, like tendon healing, occurs in a series of overlapping phases, including inflammation, proliferation, and remodeling. These events are also

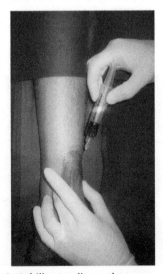

Fig. 3. PRP injection for chronic Achilles tendinopathy.

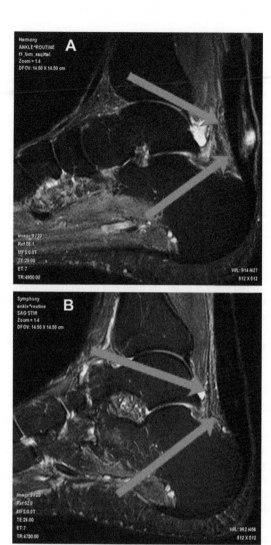

Fig. 4. Achilles MRI before and after PRP treatment. (*A*) MRI before PRP injection, partial Achilles tendon tear. (*B*) MRI 4 mo after PRP, healing of partial tear.

coordinated by growth factors and cell-to-cell interactions. Healing is dependent on local vascularity and regeneration of intramuscular nerve branches, both of which may be enhanced by PRP.[54,55] The speed of progression through these phases of healing depends on the severity of the injury and the efficiency of the patient's own biology in combination with any prescribed therapy and rehabilitation.

Despite the significance of this type of injury there are few clinical studies evaluating treatment options. Standard treatment plans attempt to decrease the bleeding and swelling associated with the injury. Recommendations include rest from activity, immediate application of ice, compressive dressings, and elevation of the affected limb. Administration of anti-inflammatory medications may alleviate pain; however, there is some evidence that this may interfere with the ability of the muscle tissue to heal. Nonsteroidal anti-inflammatory drugs may inhibit fusion of myogenic precursor

Table 3
Muscle injury grades

Grade	Tissue Damage	Symptoms
Grade 1	Few muscle fibers involved	Not apparent until conclusion of activity; very little swelling and pain only with activity
Grade 2	Moderate number of fibers involved with intact fascia	Immediately painful and moderately sore to palpation
Grade 3	Many fibers involved with incomplete fascial injury	Immediately painful and sore to palpation; patient may limp to avoid pain, severe pain with flexion vs. resistance and/or full extension
Grade 4	Complete dissociation of fibers and fascia; complete rupture	Immediate severe pain; ecchymosis below area; palpable defect

cells, thus impairing muscle healing.[56] Rehabilitation often involves a gradual return of the injured muscle to resistance exercise after the inflammatory phase has subsided. The ideal treatment for muscle injuries would accelerate the process of muscle healing while enhancing the quality of repaired tissue. The role of several growth factors in the natural repair of injured muscle is evident based on increased levels of these cytokines found in healing muscle tissue. PRP is known to contain many of these bioactive proteins.

The Role of PRP in Muscle Healing

Several growth factors within PRP have been evaluated in muscle healing. In vitro results investigating individual growth factors on skeletal muscle are variable, but certain growth factors are capable of enhancement of muscle regeneration and improved muscle force after injury.[57] Growth factors along with macrophages and the products of the COX-2 pathway regulate the inflammatory phase of skeletal muscle healing. Transforming growth factor-β1 and PGE2 may also function synergistically to balance the level of fibrosis during skeletal muscle healing.[58] In a mouse model of muscle laceration, insulin-like growth factor 1 and fibroblast growth factor-β improved muscle healing and increased fast-twitch and tetanus strength compared with controls at 1 month.[59] Autologous platelet concentrate used to treat muscle injury in a rat gastrocnemius contusion model resulted in increased satellite cell activation and myofibril width.[60] Acceleration of functional restoration was found in a human trial of elite athletes injected with ultrasound-guided PRP following muscle injury. These high-level athletes returned to sport at full strength in as early as half the expected recovery time without any evidence of excess fibrosis.[61] There are, however, no randomized controlled human studies supporting the use of PRP for muscle injuries. This is clearly an area that needs further in vitro and in vivo investigation. A prospective randomized trial using ultrasound-guided PRP for Grade 3 or Grade 4 injuries in elite athletes with return to play as an end point would provide helpful information.

DISCUSSION AND FUTURE CONSIDERATIONS

Athletes of all types are presently dissatisfied with their treatment options for tendon and muscle injuries. They are requesting better and less invasive methods to enhance or accelerate healing. Biologic options include the use of stem cells, gene therapy, and autologous or bioengineered cytokines. However, all of these possibilities are currently experimental and are not available for clinical use. Growth factors, in the form of PRP, meet many of the criteria for the ideal biologic treatment. PRP is made from the patient's own blood, which makes rejection or an adverse reaction unlikely. It can also be prepared immediately at the point of care, which makes it simple and less expensive than stem cell therapies, which often require a period of sorting and culturing before clinical use.

The exact mechanisms by which PRP initiates cellular and tissue changes are presently being investigated. It is clear that PRP induces proliferation of a variety of cell types.[38,62] PRP has also been found to recruit reparative cells.[48] This helps explain why a single PRP application can have a lasting effect on the healing process. Through interaction with macrophages, PRP may control the inflammatory reaction and thus improve tissue healing and regeneration. It is clear from in vitro studies that PRP initially inhibits IL-1 production from macrophages and reduces their proliferation. By day 4, however, this inhibition turns to stimulation of IL-1 and macrophage division.[39] This initial suppression of macrophage activity may prevent the excessive early inflammation that can lead to dense scar tissue formation. It may further be possible for PRP to regenerate tissue phenotypically closer to normal tendon and muscle by stimulating quiescent stem cells.[42] This has yet to be evaluated but should be investigated. Finally, investigating specific gene expression patterns in vitro and in vivo will contribute to a more detailed understanding of the mechanism of action of PRP.

The foregoing hypothesis supports the following one of how PRP may regenerate tendon or muscle function. PRP is applied in an unactivated form that becomes activated by the collagen within connective tissue. The PRP then releases its growth factors and cytokines. These bioactive proteins in turn stimulate local stem cells and enhance extracellular matrix gene expression. Recruitment of reparative cells from the local circulation or bone marrow then occurs. Simultaneously, PRP inhibits excess inflammation, apoptosis, and metalloproteinase activity. These interactive pathways may result in the restoration of tendon or muscle tissue, which can withstand loading with work or sports activity, thereby diminishing pain. PRP may also modulate the microvascular environment or alter efferent or afferent neural receptors. Much more investigation is required to verify the mechanism(s) of action of PRP.

Clinical investigation of PRP for tendon and muscle injuries and disorders is just beginning. There are only a few small, nonrandomized trials supporting the use of PRP for tendinosis or acute tendon tears.[9,10] Virtually no published evidence supports the use of PRP for muscle injuries in human clinical trials. Basic science data, however, point to a theoretical value. Fortunately, several prospective, double-blind randomized trials have been initiated for both tendon and muscle injuries. The results of these trials will guide future treatment recommendations.

As we look forward to these trials, it will be important to evaluate the inclusion and exclusion criteria rigorously. Defining the best types of tendon and muscle problems to treat with PRP will be a difficult but important task. The anatomic location of the injury may also be salient. For example, tendons have 3 distinct zones: the myotendinous junction, the midsubstance, and the osseotendinous junction. PRP most likely affects these zones differently. This has yet to be studied. The dosage and type of PRP employed, clearly, will also be critical elements for further study. Presently, there are proprietary PRP formulations and equipment to produce it. Standardized dosing and composition will be required to compare results. In addition, the value of ultrasound or other guidance mechanisms for injection need to be investigated. Finally, post-procedure protocols and rehabilitation methods must be coordinated to produce the best overall outcomes. For example, it may be better to gently load the tendon in the first few weeks to enhance healing.[63]

The tendon injuries that may be improved using PRP include, but are not limited to, repairs of Achilles, patellar, quadriceps, or rotator cuff tendon tears. Chronic tendinosis of any tendon may also benefit. Specifically, it could be possible to treat an acute Achilles tendon tear nonoperatively using a PRP injection. Careful evaluation will be required to determine if the rerupture rate and the tendon strength are equivalent to operative repair, without the increased risk of infection and wound complications that accompany surgical repair. Acute muscle injuries treated with hematoma aspiration and PRP injection may be another potential indication. A study of this type of injury in elite athletes has been initiated at the authors' institution.

SUMMARY

In summary, PRP has emerged as a promising, but not proven, treatment option for tendon and muscle injuries and disorders. Basic science and animal investigation have begun to help in understanding the mechanism by which PRP affects tissue restoration. Because PRP is autologous and is prepared at the point of care, it also has an excellent safety profile. It may have the ability to transform the care of muscle and tendon injuries in both elite and recreational athletes. Well-designed prospective randomized trials will be required to best understand how, when, and where to use PRP most effectively.

REFERENCES

1. The burden of musculoskeletal diseases in the United States. Source: medical expenditures panel survey, Agency for Healthcare and Quality, U.S. Department of Health and Human services, 1996–2004.
2. Knighton DR, Hunt TK, Thakral KK, et al. Role of platelets and fibrin in the healing sequence: an in vivo study of angiogenesis and collagen synthesis. Ann Surg 1982;196(4):379–88.
3. Dallari D, Savarino L, Stagni C, et al. Enhanced tibial osteotomy healing with use of bone grafts supplemented with platelet gel or platelet gel and bone marrow stromal cells. J Bone Joint Surg Am 2007;89:2413–20.
4. Carreon L, Glassman S, Anekstein Y, et al. Platelet gel (AGF) fails to increase fusion rates in instrumented posterolateral fusions. Spine 2005;30:E243–6 [discussion: E247].
5. Ranly DM, Lohmann CH, Andreacchio D, et al. Platelet-rich plasma inhibits demineralized bone matrix-induced bone formation in nude mice. J Bone Joint Surg Am 2007;89:139–47.
6. Weiner BK, Walker M. Autologous growth factors and lumbar intertransverse fusions. Spine 2003;28:1968–70 [discussion: 1971].
7. Jenis LG, Banco RJ, Kwon B. A prospective study of autologous growth factors (AGF) in lumbar interbody fusion. Spine J 2006;6(1):14–20 [E pub 2005 Dec 6].
8. Kitoh H, Kitakoji T, Tsuchiya H, et al. Distraction osteogenesis of the lower extremity with achondroplasia/hypochondroplasia treated with transplantation of culture-expanded bone marrow cells and platelet-rich plasma. J Pediatr Orthop 2007;27: 629–34.
9. Mishra A, Pavelko T. Treatment of chronic elbow tendinosis with buffered platelet-rich plasma. Am J Sports Med 2006;34:1774–8.
10. Sanchez M, Anitua E, Azofra J, et al. Comparison of surgically repaired Achilles tendon tears using platelet-rich fibrin matrices. Am J Sports Med 2007;35: 245–51.

11. Marx R. Platelet rich plasma (PRP): what is PRP and what is not PRP? Implant Dent 2001;10:225–8.

12. Horsburgh CR Jr, Clark RA, Kirkpatrick CH. Lymphokines and platelets promote human monocyte adherence to fibrinogen and fibronectin in vitro. J Leukoc Biol 1987;41(1):14–24.

13. Bielecki TM, Gazdzik TS, Arendt J, et al. Antibacterial effect of autologous platelet gel enriched with growth factors and other active substances: an in vitro study. J Bone Joint Surg Br 2007;89(3):417–20.

14. Moojem DJ, Everts PA, Schure RM, et al. Antimicrobial activity of platelet-leukocyte gel against Staphyloccus aureus. J Orthop Res 2008;26:404–10.

15. Fufa D, Shealy B, Jacobson M, et al. Activation of platelet-rich plasma using soluble Type I collagen. J Oral Maxillofac Surg 2008;66:684–90.

16. Rodeo S. Biologic augmentation of rotator cuff tendon repair. J Shoulder Elbow Surg 2007;16(Suppl 5):S191–7.

17. Liu Y, Kalén A, Risto O, et al. Fibroblast proliferation due to exposure to a platelet concentrate in vitro is pH dependent. Wound Repair Regen 2002;10(5):336–40.

18. Borzini P, Mazzucco I. Platelet-rich plasma (PRP) and platelet derivatives for topical therapy. What is true from the biologic view point? ISBT Science Series 2007; 2(1):272–81.

19. Eppley BL, Woodell JE, Higgins J. Platelet quantification and growth factor analysis from platelet rich plasma: implications for wound healing. Plast Reconstr Surg 2004;114:1502–8.

20. Everts PA, Jakimowicz JJ, van Beek M, et al. Reviewing the structural features of autologous platelet-leukocyte gel and suggestions for use in surgery. Eur Surg Res 2007;39:199–207.

21. Eppley BL, Pietrzak WS, Blanton M. Platelet-rich plasma: a review of biology and applications in plastic surgery [review]. Plast Reconstr Surg 2006;118(6): 147e–59e.

22. Hope M, Saxby TS. Tendon healing. Foot Ankle Clin 2007;12(4):553–67.

23. Awad AS, Huang L, Ye H, et al. Adenosine A2A receptor activation attenuates inflammation and injury in diabetic nephropathy. Am J Physiol Renal Physiol 2006;290(4):F828–37 [Epub 2005 Dec 6].

24. Cronstein BM. Adenosine receptors and wound healing, revised. ScientificWorldJournal 2006;6:984–91.

25. Németh ZH, Lutz CS, Csóka B, et al. Adenosine augments IL-10 production by macrophages through an A2B receptor-mediated posttranscriptional mechanism. J Immunol 2005;175(12):8260–70.

26. Cruz CM, Rinna A, Forman HJ, et al. ATP activates a reactive oxygen species-dependent oxidative stress response and secretion of proinflammatory cytokines in macrophages. J Biol Chem 2007;282(5):2871–9 [Epub 2006 Nov 27].

27. Parratt JR, West GB. Release of 5-hydroxytryptamine and histamine from tissues of the rat. J Physiol 1957;137:179–92.

28. Los G, De Weger RA, Van den Berg DT, et al. Macrophage infiltration in tumors and tumor-surrounding tissue: influence of serotonin and sensitized lymphocytes. Cancer Immunol Immunother 1988;26(2):145–52.

29. Sternberg EM, Trial J, Parker CW. Effect of serotonin on murine macrophages: suppression of Ia expression by serotonin and its reversal by 5-HT2 serotonergic receptor antagonists. J Immunol 1986;137(1):276–82.

30. Majno G, Gilmore V, Leventhal M. On the mechanism of vascular leakage caused by histaminetype mediators. A microscopic study in vivo. Circ Res 1967;21(6): 833–47.

31. Lansdown AB. Calcium: a potential central regulator in wound healing in the skin. [review]. Wound Repair Regen 2002;10(5):271–85.

32. Nho SJ, Yadav H, Shindle MK, et al. Rotator cuff degeneration: etiology and pathogenesis. Am J Sports Med 2008;36(5):987–93 [Epub 2008 Apr 15].

33. Khaliq Y, Zhanel GG. Fluoroquinolone-associated tendinopathy: a critical review of the literature [review]. Clin Infect Dis 2003;36(11):1404–10 [Epub 2003 May 20].

34. Xu Y, Murrell GA. The basic science of tendinopathy. Clin Orthop Relat Res 2008; 466(7):1528–38.

35. Wang JH, Iosifidis MI, Fu FH. Biomechanical basis for tendinopathy. Clin Orthop Relat Res 2006;443:320–32.

36. Sharma P, Maffulli N. Tendon injury and tendinopathy: healing and repair [review]. J Bone Joint Surg Am 2005;87(1):187–202.

37. Würgler-Hauri CC, Dourte LM, Baradet TC, et al. Temporal expression of 8 growth factors in tendon-to-bone healing in a rat supraspinatus model. J Shoulder Elbow Surg 2007;16(Suppl 5):S198–203.

38. Lucarelli E, Beccheroni A, Donati D, et al. Platelet-derived growth factors enhance proliferation of human stromal stem cells. Biomaterials 2003;24(18): 3095–100.

39. Woodall JR, Tucci M, Mishra A, et al. Cellular effects of platelet rich plasma: a study on HL-60 macrophage-like cells. Biomed Sci Instrum 2007;43:266–71.

40. Woodall J Jr, Mishra A, Tucci M, et al. Cellular Effects of Platelet Rich Plasma: Interleukin-1 release from PRP treated macrophage cells. Biomed Sci Instrum 2008;44:489–94.

41. Kawamura S, Ying L, Kim HJ, et al. Macrophages accumulate in the early phase of tendon-bone healing. J Orthop Res 2005;23(6):1425–32 [Epub 2005 Aug 19].

42. Bi Y, Ehirchiou D, Kilts TM, et al. Identification of tendon stem/progenitor cells and the role of the extracellular matrix in their niche. Nat Med 2007;13(10):1219–27 [Epub 2007 Sep 9].

43. Schnabel LV, Mohammed HO, Miller BJ, et al. Platelet rich plasma (PRP) enhances anabolic gene expression patterns in flexor digitorum superficialis tendons. J Orthop Res 2007;25(2):230–40.

44. de Mos M, van der Windt A, Jahr H, et al. Can platelet-rich plasma enhance tendon repair? A cell culture study. Am J Sports Med 2008;36(6):1171–8.

45. Anitua E, Sanchez M, Nurden AT, et al. Reciprocal actions of platelet-secreted TGF-beta1 on the production of VEGF and HGF by human tendon cells. Plast Reconstr Surg 2007;119:950–9.

46. Aspenberg P, Virchenko O. Platelet concentrate injection improves Achilles tendon repair in rats. Acta Orthop Scand 2004;75:93–9.

47. Virchenko O, Aspenberg P. How can one platelet injection after tendon injury lead to a stronger tendon after 4 weeks? Interplay between early regeneration and mechanical stimulation. Acta Orthop Scand 2006;77:806–12.

48. Kajikawa Y, Morihara T, Sakamoto H, et al. Platelet-rich plasma enhances the initial mobilization of circulation-derived cells for tendon healing. J Cell Physiol 2008;215:837–45.

49. Randelli P, Arrigoni P, Cabitza P, et al. Autologous platelet rich plasma for arthroscopic rotator cuff repair. A pilot study. Disabil Rehabil 2008;00:1–6.

50. Gamradt SC, Rodeo SA, Warren RF. Platelet rich plasma in rotator cuff repair. Tech Orthop Surg 2007;22:26–33.

51. Gosen T, Sluimer J. Prospective randomized study on the effect of autologous platelets injection in lateral epicondylitis compared with corticosteroid injection.

Poster presented at: 13th Congress of the European Society of Sports Traumatology, Knee Surgery and Arthroscopy (ESSKA); May 21–24, 2008; Porto, Portugal. Poster P25–444.

52. Jarvinen TA, Jarvinen TL, Kaariainen M, et al. Muscle injuries: biology and treatment. Am J Sports Med 2005;33(5):745–64.
53. Ryan AJ. Quadriceps strain, rupture, and Charlie horse. Med Sci Sports 1969;1: 106–11.
54. Yokota K, Ishida O, Sunagawa T, et al. Platelet-rich plasma accelerated surgical angiogenesis in vascular-implanted necrotic bone: an experimental study in rabbits. Acta Orthop 2008;79(1):106–10.
55. Sariguney Y, Yavuzer R, Elmas C, et al. Effect of platelet-rich plasma on peripheral nerve regeneration. J Reconstr Microsurg 2008;24(3):159–67.
56. Shen W, Prisk V, Li Y, et al. Inhibited skeletal muscle healing in cyclooxygenase-2 gene-deficient mice: the role of PGE2 and PGF2alpha. J Appl Phys 2006;101(4): 1215–21.
57. Kasemkijwattana C, Menetrey J, Bosch P, et al. Use of growth factors to improve muscle healing after strain injury. Clin Orthop Relat Res 2000;370:272–85.
58. Shen W, Li Y, Zhu J, et al. Interaction between macrophages, TGF-beta1, and the COX-2 pathway during inflammatory phase of skeletal muscle healing after injury. J Cell Physiol 2008;214(2):405–12.
59. Menetrey J, Kasemkijwattana C, Day C, et al. Growth factors improve muscle healing in vivo. J Bone Joint Surg Br 2000;82-B:131–7.
60. Wright-Carpenter T, Opolon P, Appell J, et al. Treatment of muscle injuries by local administration of autologous conditioned serum: animal experiments using a muscle contusion model. Int J Sports Med 2004;25:582–7.
61. Sanchez M, Anitua E, Andia I. Application of autologous growth factors on skeletal muscle healing. Regmed 2005. Poster Presentation. Available at: http://regmed2005.abstract-management.de/overview/?ID=314. Accessed May 15, 2008.
62. Vogel JP, Szalay K, Geiger F, et al. Platelet-rich plasma improves expansion of human mesenchymal stem cells and retains differentiation capacity and in vivo bone formation in calcium phosphate. Platelets 2006;17:462–9.
63. Aspenberg P. Stimulation of tendon repair: mechanical loading, GDFs and platelets. A mini-review. Int Orthop 2007;31(6):783–9 [Epub 2007 Jun].

New Techniques in Allograft Tissue Processing

Suketu Vaishnav, MD[a], C. Thomas Vangsness, Jr., MD[b,*],
Ryan Dellamaggiora, MD[b]

KEYWORDS

- Allograft • Processing • Sterilization
- Infection • Tissue banks

With the increased reliance on tissue allografts in orthopedic surgery and sports medicine for reconstructive procedures, the clinical safety of these implants with respect to prevention of infection and disease transmission must be ensured. According to data from the American Association of Tissue Banks (AATB), a voluntary accreditation organization that sets standards for tissue banking, approximately 1.5 million bone and tissue allografts are distributed each year by AATB-accredited tissue banks in the United States.[1] To keep up with the increasing demand of these products, the number of donors has increased to an estimated 22,000 in 2005.[2]

There have been multiple reports in the literature documenting disease transmission using connective tissue allografts.[3,4] The potential for viral and bacterial transmission is of primary concern. Specific infectious etiologies of concern include human immunodeficiency virus (HIV), hepatitis B virus (HBV) and hepatitis C virus (HCV), West Nile virus, various bacteria, and prions.

In order to improve allograft safety, tissue banks have focused attention not only on improved sterilization processes, but also on better donor screening and testing methods. In conjunction with recent guidelines and recommendations made by various regulatory bodies, such as the Centers for Disease Control and Prevention (CDC) and Food and Drug Administration (FDA), tissue banks are hoping to decrease the actual and theoretic risk of disease transmission.

There is great concern regarding allograft safety within the orthopedic community. In a 2006 survey performed by the American Orthopaedic Society for Sports Medicine (AOSSM), allograft use and concerns were explored among its membership.[5,6] More

[a] Department of Orthopaedic Surgery, University of Southern California, Keck School of Medicine, LAC+USC Medical Center, 1200 N. State Street, GNH 3900, Los Angeles, CA 90033, USA
[b] Department of Orthopaedic Surgery, University of Southern California, Keck School of Medicine, Healthcare Consultation Center, 1520 San Pablo Street, Suite 2000, Los Angeles, CA 90033-4608, USA
* Corresponding author.
E-mail address: vangsnes@usc.edu (C. Thomas Vangsness).

Clin Sports Med 28 (2009) 127–141
doi:10.1016/j.csm.2008.08.002
0278-5919/08/$ – see front matter © 2008 Elsevier Inc. All rights reserved.

sportsmed.theclinics.com

than 85% of respondents indicated the use of allografts in reconstructive procedures. Even though more than 75% of members reported using allografts from AATB-accredited tissue banks, about half of all respondents (46%) were not certain whether the tissues were sterilized or did not know the specific sterilization process used. There was also a consensus regarding the need for stricter regulations and more randomized clinical studies examining existing sterilization methods.

As a result of complications associated with allograft contamination, concern among the general public regarding allograft sterilization techniques and safety has increased. As a consequence, federal supervision of allograft processing has resulted in strict standards for tissue preparation and processing by tissue banks. In addition, independent oversight organizations such as the AATB have aided this effort.

To appreciate the realistic risks involved in using connective tissue allografts, it is important to know which infectious etiologies have been historically transmitted, the current donor screening and testing methods utilized, and the various sterilization guidelines and processes currently employed by various tissue preparers.

HISTORICAL INFECTION TRANSMISSION
Viral Infection

HIV, HBV, HCV, and human T-lymphotropic virus (HTLV) have all been transmitted by tissue transplantation.[7–9] In a 2004 study evaluating viremia rates among tissue donors in the United States, the prevalence of confirmed positive tests among tissue donors was 0.093% for anti-HIV, 0.22% for HBsAg, 1.091% for anti-HCV, and 0.068% for anti-HTLV.[10] The estimated probability of viremia at the time of donation was 1 in 55,000, 1 in 34,000, 1 in 42,000, and 1 in 128,000, respectively. The authors concluded that the prevalence rates of HBV, HCV, HIV, and HTLV infections are lower among tissue donors than in the general population. However, the estimated probability of undetected viremia at the time of tissue donation is higher among tissue donors than among first-time blood donors.

The first reported case of HIV infection through bone transplantation occurred in 1988.[11] Since then, there have been multiple documented cases in the literature of HIV transmission worldwide through bone and other connective tissues.[12–15] It should be noted however, that many of these transmissions occurred before the implementation of extensive donor screening for viruses and bacteria or the availability of validated serologic tests.[16]

HCV has also been recently implicated in disease transmission during patellar tendon-bone allograft use. In June 2002, the CDC reported the transmission of HCV from a donor whose serum at the time of death in October 2002 had no detectable antibodies to HCV (anti-HCV).[8] The ensuing investigation conducted by the CDC and the local Department for Health Services (DHS) confirmed that the donor was HCV RNA-positive and the probable source of HCV infection. Further inquiries showed that the donor was the cause of HCV transmission for at least 8 other organ and tissue recipients.

In 1991, transmission of HTLV was reported in Sweden after the living donor first contracted the virus through a blood transfusion during hip surgery 4 years earlier.[17] A subsequent hip surgery resulted in donation of an infected femoral head allograft, which eventually led to infection in the recipient.

Bacterial Infection

Bacterial infection associated with musculoskeletal allograft use is a relatively rare event according to the CDC. In a March 2002 report, the CDC noted that 26 allograft-associated bacterial infections had been identified over the preceding 5 years.[18]

In November 2001, a 23-year-old male underwent reconstructive knee surgery at a hospital in Minnesota using a femoral condyle allograft. Three days after surgery, he developed signs and symptoms consistent with infection at the surgical site. The patient subsequently progressed to shock and died. Blood cultures taken before death grew *Clostridium sordellii*. A second individual in Illinois received a fresh frozen femoral condyle and meniscus allograft from the same donor. This individual developed septic arthritis. There was no evidence that showed the donor was septic or had risk factors for *Clostridium* infection. Seven additional patients received tissue from the same donor, but none developed infection.[18]

Of the 26 reports received by the CDC (**Table 1**), 13 (50%) were of patients infected with *Clostridium* spp. (*C. septicum*,[12] *C. sordellii*[1]). Of these patients 11 (85%) received tissue processed by the same tissue bank. This tissue bank has been identified in subsequent news reports as CryoLife (Kennesaw, GA).[19,20]

A December 2003 report by the CDC highlighted the case of a 17-year-old male who underwent anterior cruciate reconstructive surgery with the use of patellar tendon-bone allograft and subsequently became infected with *Streptococcus Pyogenes* (group A streptococcus, [GAS]).[21] The patient was treated with allograft removal with irrigation and debridement in addition to antibiotic treatment. Blood, wound, and aspirate cultures all grew GAS. Five other patients received allografts from the same donor, but no other adverse outcomes resulted.

According to the CDC, cultures of the donor's tissues, obtained by the tissue recovery organization before distribution to 2 tissue processors, yielded GAS. Preprocessing cultures obtained by the tissue processor also yielded GAS. The allografts were then processed using aseptic technique and an antimicrobial solution, but no sterilization procedure (eg, gamma irradiation) was used. After the recovered tissues were processed, all post-processing cultures were reported as negative, and these allografts were distributed.

The use of aseptic recovery techniques and processing attempts to minimize contamination of donor tissue. This however, does not guarantee elimination of contamination from the donor or recovery process. Furthermore, AATB-accredited tissue processors adhere to a maximum allowable tissue recovery time period after asystole. Failure to adhere to these standards can result in contaminated donor tissue and an increased possibility of an infected tissue allograft.[4,16] Overall concerns about infections exist with respect to microbes present in the cadaveric tissue itself in

Table 1
Allograft-associated infections investigated by CDC transmitted by musculoskeletal grafts[16]

	Clostridium Spp	Other Infections
Tendons for anterior cruciate ligament	8	10
Femoral condyles	2	1
Bone	2	1
Meniscus	1	1
Total	13	13

Note. Not all of these were probably associated or proven to be associated with the allograft; they were possibly associated with the allograft.

Data from Vangsness CT Jr., Wagner PP, Moore TM, et al. Overview of safety issues concerning the preparation and processing of soft-tissue allografts. Arthroscopy 2006;22(12):1351–8.

addition to exogenous contamination with microorganisms during the harvesting or processing of the tissue.

CURRENT REGULATIONS AND GUIDELINES
Governmental Regulations

Human cells or tissue intended for implantation, transplantation, infusion, or transfer into a human recipient is regulated as a human cell, tissue, and cellular and tissue-based product or HCT/P. The Center for Biologics Evaluation and Research (CBER) regulates HCT/Ps under 21 Code of Federal Regulations (CFR) Parts 1270 and 1271.[22] In May 2005, FDA implemented its requirements for Current Good Tissue Practice (CGTP) for organizations that manufacture HCT/Ps.[23]

These regulations require tissue establishments to screen and test donors, to prepare and follow written procedures for the prevention of the spread of communicable disease (eg, viruses, bacteria, fungi, parasites, and transmissible spongiform encephalopathy agents), and to maintain records. FDA has published 3 final rules to broaden the scope of products subject to regulation and to include more comprehensive requirements to prevent the introduction, transmission, and spread of communicable disease.

One final rule requires firms to register and list their HCT/Ps with FDA. The second rule requires tissue establishments to evaluate donors, through screening and testing, to reduce the transmission of infectious diseases through tissue transplantation. The third and final rule establishes current good tissue practices for HCT/Ps. FDA's revised regulations are contained in Part 1271 and apply to tissues recovered after May 25, 2005.[22,23]

The FDA does not specifically require that recovered tissue undergo sterilization. In addition, it does not require that recovery and processing occur in an aseptic manner. It does, however, mandate that any written representation that an establishment's processing methods reduce the risk of transmission of communicable diseases by an allograft, including a representation of sterility or pathogen inactivation, must be based on a fully verified or validated process.[6,16] Supervision of tissue processors is performed through mandated federal and state regulations. As of March 2007, FDA and 5 states require licensing; these include New York, Florida, California, Georgia, and Maryland.[16,23–25]

The tissue processor is responsible for making a donor-eligibility determination. This is a conclusion that a donor is either eligible or ineligible to donate cells or tissues to be used in an HCT/P, based on the results of donor screening. A donor is eligible only if (1) screening shows that the donor is free from risk factors for, and clinical evidence of, infection due to relevant communicable disease agents and diseases and (2) test results for relevant communicable disease agents are negative or nonreactive.

FDA guidelines require that all donor tissue be screened for HIV types 1 and 2, HBV, HCV, *Trepenoma pallidum*, and human transmissible spongiform encephalopathies. As of August 2007, FDA mandates that donor tissue must also be negative for HIV-1 nucleic acid testing (NAT), HCV NAT, and HBV core antibody. NAT screening uses a highly sensitive polymerase chain reaction test to look for viral genetic material, which greatly improves safety.

Furthermore, it is the responsibility of the tissue processor to maintain adequate and detailed records documenting the type of tissue being processed, the collecting organization that recovered the tissue, the tests performed on the tissue and their results, processing steps, and the destination of the tissue. Records pertaining to a particular HCT/P must be retained for at least 10 years after the date of its administration. This includes records created by laboratories performing donor eligibility testing. In addition, the tissue must be distinctly labeled with an identification code linking it to the donor.

The Joint Commission

Formerly known as the Joint Commission on Accreditation of Health care Organizations (JCAHO), the Joint Commission is a regulatory entity independent of FDA. Effective August 6, 2007, the Joint Commission enforced its most recent set of Tissue Storage and Issuance Standards.[23] The Tissue Storage and Issuance standards apply to human and nonhuman cellular-based implantable and transplantable products. These standards dictate that the source facility should be registered with FDA and licensed by the state, if the state in which the implanting organization resides requires licensure.

The standards call for organizations to develop procedures to address the critical areas of tissue acquisition and storage, record keeping and tracking, and adverse events/infection follow-up. Written procedures must cover steps describing the tissue: ordering, receipt, storage (includes temperature monitoring and recording, requirements for storage equipment alarms, and backup plans), handling, preparation for use, tracking (from receipt, through storage, and to the recipient), and handling of possible or proven adverse events, and recalls.

The organization will need to be able to trace the chain of events related to implanted tissue for both reporting and investigational purposes. According to the Joint Commission standards, records should permit bidirectional tracing of any tissue to report potential disease transmission to the recipient when notified by the donor source facility, report adverse patient reactions to the donor source facility, and investigate the chain of events of such activities. All records are required to be kept for a minimum of 10 years from the latest date of tissue transplantation, distribution, or expiration.

Nongovernmental Agencies

The AATB was founded in 1976 as a not-for-profit organization designed to spread voluntary safety standards and ensure that human tissues intended for transplantation are safe and free of infectious disease, of uniform high quality, and available in quantities sufficient to meet national needs.[26] The organization comprises nearly 100 accredited tissue banks and 1,100 individual members.

In 1984, the AATB published its *Standards for Tissue Banking*. Most recently updated and revised, the 12th edition was published in 2008. In 1986, the AATB initiated a mandatory Accreditation Program for its institutional members to ensure that tissue-banking activities are performed in compliance with these standards. In 1988, the AATB began a certification program for individuals working in tissue banking. AATB accreditation is based on compliance with standards relating to donor eligibility criteria, retrieval, processing, storage and distribution, and record keeping of transplantable human tissues. Banks are inspected and given a renewal of accreditation every 3 years.

In March 2005, the AATB initiated NAT screening for HIV and HCV. NAT screening significantly improves the ability to identify viral infected tissue by decreasing the window period, which prevents detection by methods using antibody testing alone. As mentioned previously, NAT screening is now required as part of FDA regulations as of August 2007.

With respect to culture results, AATB requires that any positive final culture will result in discarding the processed allograft unless an allograft rework protocol has been validated to eliminate the organism identified. Furthermore, the AATB has required the discarding of any allograft that cultures positive (preprocessing) for Clostridium or S pyogenes (GAS).[4,6]

It is estimated that more than 90% of musculoskeletal tissues in the United States are distributed by AATB-accredited tissue banks. Current membership includes 104 accredited tissue banks.

Other organizations involved in monitoring and ensuring allograft safety are the AABB (formerly know as the American Association of Blood Banks) and the International Organization for Standardization (ISO). The AABB recently published their Guidelines for Managing Tissue Allografts in Hospitals—a document closely following Joint Commission requirements in content and structure.

ALLOGRAFT PREPARATION AND PROCESSING
Donor Screening

Efforts to ensure allograft safety begin with screening, which involves an exhaustive donor screening process scrutinizing the source from which the allograft is procured. In addition to reviewing medical records, a medical history and social risk assessment are obtained by interviewing surviving relatives, hospitals, and clinics. If available, information from previous blood donation can be used. Autopsy reports (if performed) can provide additional insight as to the donor's risk factors for infectious diseases.

Testing required by FDA and AATB will decrease the likelihood of releasing tissue from a donor with a viral infection. This, however, is limited by the window period associated with current testing procedures—the time frame without detectable antibodies or antigens.[27] NAT decreases this phase to about 7 days for HIV and HCV infections and 8 days for HBV infection. Due to the greater prevalence of HCV and HBV than that of HIV, the risk of contracting HIV by way of tissue allograft implantation is lower than that for HBV and HCV. Current screening and testing protocols have placed the risk of implanting tissue from an HIV-infected donor to as low as 1 in 1 million.[28,29] The current risk of transmitting HCV from unprocessed tissue that is HCV negative is estimated to be 1 in 421,000.[10]

Human errors in screening and processing must also be taken into consideration. Data from blood donation gives insight into allograft-associated bacterial infection risk. The risk of bacterial infection from fresh platelet infusion is reported to be between 1 in 2000 to 1 in 5000.[27,30,31]

The incidence of postoperative orthopedic infection rates ranges from 0.6% to 6.6% according to the National Nosocomial Infection Surveillance System of the CDC.[32] True incidence rates regarding the risk of infection from transplanted allograft tissue are not known, but such events are likely underreported and are difficult to confirm. However, there were 19 published reports during a 5-year period during which approximately 4 to 5 million tissues were distributed.[33] Although a precise incidence number is not meaningful given the lack of an accurate detection system, the rate of transmission is around 1 confirmed event in every few hundred thousand allografts implanted. This rate of recognized reported infection is approximately 2 orders of magnitude lower than that with solid organs, but the absolute number of tissue-related infections may make this risk more significant given the millions of allograft tissues implanted compared with the thousands of organ transplants annually. However, the current risk of an allograft-transmitted infection to most patients appears to be much less than the overall risk of perioperative nosocomial infection and should be put into appropriate perspective.[6]

Tissue Processing

Tissue processing begins when the allograft tissue is recovered under aseptic conditions to minimize the amount of contamination to the procured tissue. This is usually performed under standard, sterile operating room techniques. The tissue is collected by a surgical team of technicians using sterile technique in addition to prepping and draping of the procurement site. The collected tissue is then cultured, packaged under sterile conditions, labeled, and shipped in specified containers under wet ice temperatures. Even though the tissue may be procured under aseptic conditions, it should not be considered sterile. As stated in the CDC's Morbidity and Mortality Weekly Report from March 15, 2002, "aseptically processed tissue should not be considered sterile, and health care providers should be informed of the possible risk for bacterial infection."[18] Contamination can occur both through the patient's own gastrointestinal or respiratory tracts in addition to that introduced by handling of the tissue by health care workers. This contamination is reduced but not completely eliminated using antibiotic solution washing.[34,35]

Culturing of aseptically harvested tissue provides limited information because studies have shown that only 78% to 92% of these cultures are accurate in identifying bacterial or fungal contamination.[36] Furthermore, the United States Pharmacopeial Convention specifically states that cultures for sterility can only be used to monitor a previously validated sterilization process and should not be used as definitive evidence of sterilization.[37]

Tissue Disinfection

The process of removing any possible contamination from the allograft tissue is defined as disinfection. Sterilization refers to the process of inactivating or killing all forms of life, especially microbes.[38] Due to the complex three-dimensional nature of musculoskeletal tissue, standard sterilization techniques employed on metals and plastics cannot be used without permanently compromising its biologic and structural properties. Furthermore, varying tissue absorptive properties also make it difficult for disinfectants to effectively penetrate the allograft tissue and be successfully washed out. In order for the sterilization process to be effective, it must rid the tissue of pathogens without altering tissue biomechanical characteristics or tertiary collagen structure.

The effectiveness of sterilization methods is assessed as the sterility assurance level (SAL). This expression measures the likelihood that a viable pathogen exists on a sterilized graft. Currently, FDA requires implantable medical devices to have an SAL of 10^{-3}, meaning there is a 1 in 1000 probability that a live microorganism exists on the sterilized product. It should be noted, however, that many tissue banks attempt to reach an SAL of 10^{-6} for processed allografts, the level recommended by the Association for the Advancement of Medical Instrumentation and required by the AATB.[39–42] This however, must not compromise the structural or functional integrity of the device. Both FDA and AATB require tissue banks to support any written claims they make regarding the effectiveness of sterilization of tissue allografts with verified and validated processes.[6,16,22,23]

Many different processes and protocols are employed by different tissue banks in attempts to ensure proper disinfection and sterilization of tissue allograft (**Table 2**). No standardized protocol has been shown to be superior. There are also no mandated sterilization processes required by FDA. An often complex combination of techniques under a patented protocol is used by each individual tissue bank. These include the use of irradiation, soaking and washing with chemical and antibiotic reagents, and

Table 2
Comparison between aseptic processing, ethylene oxide, gamma irradiation, and chemical soaking methods and their sterilization abilities and properties[16]

	Aseptic Processing	Ethylene Oxide	Gamma Irradiation	Chemical Soaking
Kills bacteria	No	Yes	Yes	Yes
Kills fungi	No	Yes	Yes	Yes
Kills spores	No	Yes	Yes	No
Kills enveloped and non-enveloped viruses (eg, HIV, hepatitis A)	No	Yes	Yes (dose-dependent)	No
Removes blood and lipids	Surface only	No	No	Surface only
Preserves strength	Yes	Yes	Decreases (dose-dependent)	Yes
Preserves biocompatibility	Yes	Yes	Yes	Yes
Penetrates into tissue	Surface only	Thickness-dependent	Full penetration	Surface only

Data from Vangsness CT Jr., Wagner PP, Moore TM, et al. Overview of safety issues concerning the preparation and processing of soft-tissue allografts. Arthroscopy 2006;22(12):1351–8.

lypophilization (freeze-drying) and cryopreservation among various other techniques. This is often followed by terminal sterilization in the form of either gamma irradiation or with the use of ethylene oxide. Packaging and storage are performed according to AATB guidelines.

Gamma irradiation is a popular method used by tissue banks to sterilize recovered tissue. Traditionally, a dose of 25 kGy has been recommended. Although many tissue banks use a dose of 25 kGy, some banks use a higher dose, whereas others use a lower one. Given the concerns regarding the compromise of biomechanical properties of allografts and the possibility of premature clinical failure after undergoing this process, some tissue banks elect not to use gamma irradiation altogether. Studies performed on animal tissue have demonstrated that gamma irradiation can weaken allograft bone in an additive and dose-dependent manner.[43–45] Many studies have also been performed on human specimens demonstrating this association as well.[46–52] The mechanisms by which gamma irradiation sterilization damages allograft tissue are not well known; there is evidence that the damage is induced through free radical attack on collagen.

In efforts to reduce the structural damage caused by gamma irradiation, attempts have been made to modify this process. Recent studies have shown that the pretreatment of allograft tissues with radioprotectant scavengers is successful in blocking the activity of free radicals by reducing the extent of damage to collagen.[53,54] This has been shown to help maintain the mechanical strength of sterilized tissue, potentially improving the functional life of the allograft following implantation. The use of high-dose (50 kGy) irradiation has been tested on radioprotectant-treated cancellous bone allografts with the effects of inactivating viral pathogens including HIV and HCV. These investigators demonstrated that the ultimate compressive strength and modulus of elasticity were equal to conventionally irradiated (18 kGy) and nonirradiated control bone grafts.[55] A follow-up study performed by the same investigators on high-dose (50 kGy) irradiated semi-tendinosus tendons pretreated with a radioprotectant solution demonstrated preimplantation biomechanical properties similar to the nonirradiated and 18-kGy groups.[56]

Only a few in vivo studies have compared irradiated versus nonirradiated allografts. One such clinical study compared patients undergoing ACL reconstruction with nonirradiated Achilles allografts with those receiving irradiated (dose 2.0–2.5 mRad) Achilles allografts. The authors found an alarmingly high rate of failures (33%, 11 out of 33) in the irradiated group compared with the nonirradiated group (2.4%, 1 out of 42). These results led the author to discontinue the use of irradiated allografts during ACL surgery.[57] Another study involving bilateral ACL reconstructions in a goat model showed a similar trend. One extremity had an ACL reconstruction performed with an irradiated (4 mRad) patellar tendon allograft, whereas the other received a fresh frozen control allograft. After retrieval of allografts 6 months after surgery, the irradiated grafts showed lower stiffness and maximum force compared with controls but no differences were seen in modulus, maximum stress, or biochemical characteristics.[58]

Some companies employ the freeze-drying process of lyophilization. This process entails an initial freezing of the tissue followed by multiple steps (sublimation, desorption) to reduce the total water content to levels that will no longer support chemical or biological activity.[59,60] Studies have shown that the freeze-drying can decrease the viral load of infected musculoskeletal tissue to subinfectious levels.[12,61] However, other reports noted the inability of the process to completely inactivate HIV in a feline model.[13]

SPECIFIC PROCESSES FOR TISSUE PREPARATION

Many different patented techniques are used by tissue banks (**Table 3**), each with specific and unique steps. The goal of these techniques is to effectively eradicate and inactivate infectious microorganisms while at the same time preserving the biomechanical properties of the tissue allograft. There are no definitive studies proving that one process is more effective or efficacious. Newer techniques continue to be developed with the goal of patient safety. As such, more clinical studies will be required to validate these processes.

Regeneration Technologies (Alachua, FL) uses the Biocleanse tissue process to treat its tissue allografts. The Biocleanse process involves sterilizing tissue for 4 hours using several dozen rapidly oscillating pressure/vacuum cycles above and below atmospheric pressure. During this time, the grafts are exposed to various chemicals such as alcohol, hydrogen peroxide, detergents, and rinses. This serves to remove blood, viruses, bacteria, and spores to achieve reduced antigenicity. The processor claims an SAL of 10^{-6} with this method. Studies involving tibialis anterior and bone-patellar tendon-bone allografts treated with the Biocleanse process cite mechanical characteristics similar to irradiated and fresh-frozen controls.[62,63]

LifeNet (Virginia Beach, VA) uses the Allowash XG formula. This process incorporates both ultrasonics and centrifugation with biological reagents. When processing bone-patellar tendon-bone allografts, tissue is terminally sterilized using 13 to 18 kGy of irradiation. LifeNet claims an SAL of 10^{-6} and states that tissue properties are not adversely affected by this process.[6,16]

The Musculoskeletal Transplant Foundation (MTF, Edison, NJ) does not terminally sterilize most cancellous and cortical allografts with irradiation. Rather, a series of chemical steps using nonionic detergents, hydrogen peroxide, and alcohol is used.

Table 3
Specific sterilization methods used by specific tissue banks

Tissue Bank	Nonprofit, for Profit	Sterilization Method
RTI	For profit	BioCleanse—A validated, automated, pharmaceutical sterilization process using vacuum/pressure and chemical sterilants. The Tutoplast process comprises numerous phases as shown in the following example: 1. Lipids are removed in an ultrasonic acetone bath. 2. A series of alternating hyperosmotic saline and deionized water baths. 3. An oxidative treatment with hydrogen peroxide (H_2O_2). 4. A final acetone wash. The acetone wash, followed by vacuum extraction, dehydrates the tissue. Terminally sterilized using low-dose gamma irradiation. Yields a SAL of 10^{-6}.
LifeNet	Nonprofit	Allowash XG (An intensive decontamination and scrubbing regime) gamma irradiated, sterility validated. Validated to SAL of 10^{-6}.
MTF	Nonprofit	Allograft tissue purification process (ATP)
Community tissue services	Nonprofit	Grafts are soaked and rinsed in antibiotics, hydrogen peroxide, alcohol, sterile water, and Allowash solutions and irradiated at a dosage between 15 and –25 kGy.
Osteotech	For profit	Permeint TM Combination of ethanol and nonionic detergent.
Bone bank allograft	Nonprofit	GraftCleanse- ISO 11,137-2 Method-1 A validated sterilization process with an SAL of 10^{-6} gamma sterilized at 19.8–24.2 kGy.
Allosource	Nonprofit	Validated SterileR disinfection process plus low-dose gamma irradiation assures SAL of 10^{-6}.
TBI	Nonprofit	TranZgraft Proprietary wash plus low-temperature, low-dose gamma irradiation. A validated sterilization process with an SAL of 10^{-6}.

The MTF recovers and processes bone-patellar tendon-bone allografts and other soft tissues aseptically and processes them using gentamicin, Amphotericin B, and Primaxin. The antibiotics are subsequently washed out of the tissue at the end of processing to nondetectable levels (<1 ppm). If a high bioburden is believed to exist, some incoming tissues are pretreated with a low-dose gamma irradiation (12–18 kGy). The MTF tissue label states "aseptically processed passes USP <71> for sterility" but there are no claims that the tissue is sterile. The MTF does not terminally sterilize tissue with irradiation because of concern of detrimental effects on tissue material properties.[6]

Terminal Sterilization and Packaging

Each tissue bank employs a patented process of tissue processing and sterilization involving a multitude of specific steps. The last step in tissue processing before packaging is usually terminal sterilization. This is performed to address concerns about contamination during the handling and packaging processes. Multiple techniques exist to inactivate bacteria, spores, and viruses (**Table 2**). Traditionally, tissue banks have used one of two methods for disinfection—gamma irradiation or ethylene oxide gas (EO).[64–72] However, EO has been used with less frequency due to the concerns of host reaction with tissue treated using EO.[64,65,68]

After tissue processing and packaging are completed, the tissue allograft is usually stored frozen. Most major tissue banks follow common storage and packaging guidelines as dictated by the AATB. This includes deep-freezing at temperatures between −40 and −80 °C.[6,16]

Summary

With the increasing medical demand and dependence on allograft use in reconstructive orthopedic and sports surgery, more scrutiny has been directed toward the safety and reliability of these soft tissue allografts. Improved methods of donor screening, tissue processing and disinfection, and storage, in conjunction with closer oversight and more stringent guidelines by the CDC, FDA, and AATB, have decreased the risks of disease transmission.

Furthermore, newer patented techniques employed by tissue banks attempt to ensure cleaner tissues with greater SALs. With these new techniques arise questions not only of tissue safety, but also the maintenance of biomechanical integrity. Multiple reports have cited compromised allograft properties with certain techniques. Therefore, more clinical investigation is required before these methods can be deemed safe and reliable.

As such, it is the responsibility of the orthopedic surgeon to be familiar with the sterilization processes used for the grafts they use in reconstructive surgery. It is recommended that grafts from AATB-accredited banks be used whenever possible.

BIBLIOGRAPHY

1. Centers for Disease Control and Prevention. About tissue transplants 2006. Available at: http://www.cdc.gov/ncidod/dhqp/tissueTransplantsFAQ.html. Accessed May 22, 2008.
2. Vangsness CT Jr. Soft-tissue allograft processing controversies. J Knee Surg 2006;19:215–9.
3. Nemzek JA, Swenson CL, Arnoczky SP. Retroviral transmission by the transplantation of connective tissue allografts. An experimental study. J Bone Joint Surg Am 1994;76:1036–41.
4. Vangsness CT Jr, Garcia IA, Mills CR, et al. Allograft transplantation in the knee: tissue regulation, procurement, processing, and sterilization. Am J Sports Med 2003;31:474–81.
5. 2006 AOSSM Orthopaedic Surgical Procedure Survey on Allografts. Naperville (IL): Leever Research Services; 2006.

6. McAllister DR, Joyce MJ, Mann BJ, et al. Allograft update: the current status of tissue regulation, procurement, processing, and sterilization. Am J Sports Med 2007;35(12):2148–58.

7. Joyce MJ, Greenwald AS, Rigney R, et al. Report on musculoskeletal allograft tissue safety. Presented at the American Academy of Orthopaedic Surgeons 71st Annual Meeting, San Francisco, March 10–14, 2004.

8. Centers for Disease Control and Prevention (CDC). Hepatitis C virus transmission from an antibody-negative organ and tissue donor–United States, 2000–2002. MMWR Morb Mortal Wkly Rep 2003;52:273–4, 276.

9. Eastlund T, Strong DM. Infectious disease transmission through tissue transplantation. In: Phillips GO, editor, Advances in tissue banking, vol. 7. Singapore: World Scientific; 2004. p. 51–131.

10. Zou S, Dodd RY, Stramer SL, et al. Probability of viremia with HBV, HCV, HIV, and HTLV among tissue donors in the United States. N Engl J Med 2004;351: 751–9.

11. Centers for Disease Control and Prevention (CDC). Epidemiologic notes and reports transmission of hiv through bone transplantation: case report and public health recommendations. MMWR Morb Mortal Wkly Rep 1988;37(39):597–9.

12. Asselmeier MA, Caspari RB, Bottenfield S. A review of allograft processing and sterilization techniques and their role in transmission of the human immunodeficiency virus. Am J Sports Med 1993;21:170–5.

13. Simonds RJ, Holmberg SD, Hurwitz RL, et al. Transmission of human immunodeficiency virus type 1 from a seronegative organ and tissue donor. N Engl J Med 1992;326:726–32.

14. Simonds RJ. HIV transmission by organ and tissue transplantation. AIDS 1993; 7(Suppl 2):S35–8.

15. Li CM, Ho YR, Liu YC. Transmission of human immunodeficiency virus through bone transplantation: a case report. J Formos Med Assoc 2001;100(5):350–1.

16. Vangsness CT Jr, Wagner PP, Moore TM, et al. Overview of safety issues concerning the preparation and processing of soft-tissue allografts. Arthroscopy 2006; 22(12):1351–8.

17. Sanzen L, Carlsson A. Transmission of human T-cell lymphotrophic virus type 1 by a deep-frozen bone allograft. Acta Orthop Scand 1997;68:72–4.

18. Centers for Disease Control and Prevention (CDC). Update: Allograft-associated bacterial infections—United States, 2002. MMWR Morb Mortal Wkly Rep 2002;(51):207–10.

19. Blakeslee S. Knee ligament in a transplant leads to illness. NY Times December 5, 2003. Health section.

20. Kainer MA, Linden JV, Whaley DN, et al. Clostridium infections associated with musculoskeletal-tissue allografts. N Engl J Med 2004;350:2564–71.

21. Centers for Disease Control and Prevention (CDC). Invasive Streptococcus pyogenes after allograft implantation—Colorado, 2003. MMWR Morb Mortal Wkly Rep 2003;(52):1173–6.

22. US Food and Drug Administration. Eligibility determination for donors of human cells tissues, and cellular and tissue based products: final rule 21 CFR parts 210, 211, 820, 1271. Fed Regist 2004;69:29786–834. Available at: http://www.fda.gov/cber/rules/suitdonor.pdf. Accessed July 15, 2008.

23. US Food and Drug Administration. Current good tissue practice for human cell, tissue, and cellular and tissue-based product establishments: inspection and enforcement; final rule 21 CFR parts 16, 1270, and 1271 (D,E,F). Fed Reg 2004;document #16–611-68688. Available at: http://a257.g.akamaitech.net/7/

257/2422/06jun20041800/edocket.access.gpo.gov/2004/pdf/04-25798.pdf. Accessed July 15, 2008.

24. Patel R, Trampuz A. Infections transmitted through musculoskeletal-tissue allografts. N Engl J Med 2004;350(25):2544–6.

25. The Joint Commission: tissue storage and issuance standards. 2007. Available at: http://www.jointcommission.org/AccreditationPrograms/Hospitals/Standards/FAQs/Provision+of+Care/Tissue+Storage+Issuance/app_tsis.htm. Accessed July 15, 2008.

26. The American Association of Tissue Banks. Available at: http://www.aatb.org. Accessed July 15, 2008.

27. Dodd RY, Notari EP 4th, Stramer SL. Current prevalence and incidence of infectious disease markers and estimated window-period risk in the American red cross blood donor population. Transfusion 2002;42:975–9.

28. Buck BE, Malinin TI. Human bone and tissue allografts. Preparation and safety. Clin Orthop Relat Res 1994;8–17.

29. Gocke DJ. Tissue donor selection and safety. Clin Orthop 2005;435:17–21.

30. Fang CT, Chambers LA, Kennedy J, et al. American Red Cross Regional Blood Centers. Detection of bacterial contamination in apheresis platelet products: American Red Cross experience 2004. Transfusion 2005;(45):1845–52.

31. Strong DM, Katz L. Blood-bank testing for infectious diseases: how safe is blood transfusion? Trends Mol Med 2002;8:355–8.

32. Centers for Disease Control and Prevention. Semiannual Report of the National Nosocomial Infection Surveillance (NNIS) System. Atlanta (GA): Centers for Disease Control and Prevention, US Dept of Health and Human Services; 2000: 11–13 [tables 5 and 6].

33. Srinivasan A. Epidemiology of organ- and tissue-transmitted infections. Presented at: workshop on preventing organ- and tissue allograft-transmitted infection: priorities for public health intervention 2005; Atlanta (GA). Proceedings. Available at: http://www.cdc.gov/ncidod/dhqp/pdf/bbp/organ_tissueWorkshop_June2005.pdf. Accessed July 15, 2008.

34. Hirn MY, Salmela PM, Vuento RE. High-pressure saline washing of allografts reduces bacterial contamination. Acta Orthop Scand 2001;72:83–5.

35. Chiu CK, Lau PY, Chan SW, Fong CM, Sun LK. Microbial contamination of femoral head allografts. Hong Kong Med J 2004;10(6):401–5.

36. Veen MR, Bloem RM, Petit PL. Sensitivity and negative predictive value of swab cultures in musculoskeletal allograft procurement. Clin Orthop Relat Res 1994; 299:259–63.

37. United States Pharmacopeial Convention. Sterilization and sterility assurance of compendial articles. Chapter 1211. In: United States Pharmacopeia and National Formulary (USP 25-NF 20). Rockville (MD): United States Pharmacopeial Convention; 2002.

38. Block SS. Peroxygen compounds. In: Block SS, editor. Disinfection, sterilization, and preservation. 5th edition. Philadelphia: Lippincott, Williams & Wilkins; 2001. p. 1162.

39. ANSI/AAMI/ISO 11137-1994: Sterilization of health care products—requirements for validation and routine control—radiation sterilization. New York: American National Standards Institute; 1994.

40. Forsell JH. Irradiation of musculoskeletal tissue. In: Tomford WW, editor. Musculoskeletal tissue banking. New York: Raven Press; 1993. p. 149–80.

41. How safe are soft-tissue allografts? American Academy of Orthopaedic Surgeons. Available at: http://www.aaos.org/news/bulletin/aug07/clinical1.asp. Accessed July 15, 2008.

42. Nguyen H, Morgan DAF, Forwood MR. Sterilization of allograft bone: is 25 kGy the gold standard for gamma irradiation? Cell Tissue Bank 2007;8:81–91.
43. Pelker RR, Friedlaender GE, Markham TC, et al. Effects of freezing and freeze-drying on the biomechanical properties of rat bone. J Orthop Res 1984;1:405–11.
44. Kang JS, Kim NH. The biomechanical properties of deep freezing and freeze drying bones and their biomechanical changes after in-vivo allograft. Yonsei Med J 1995;36:332–5.
45. Pelker RR, McKay J, Troiano N, et al. Allograft incorporation: a biomechanical evaluation in a rat model. J Orthop Res 1989;7:585–9.
46. Stevenson S, Emery SE, Goldberg VM. Factors affecting bone graft incorporation. Clin Orthop 1996;324:6–74.
47. Conrad EU, Ericksen DP, Tencer AF, et al. The effects of freeze-drying and rehydration on cancellous bone. Clin Orthop 1993;290:279–84.
40. Pelker RR, Friedlaender GE, Markham TC. Biomechanical properties of bone allografts. Clin Orthop 1983;174:54–7.
49. Cornu O, Banse X, Docquier PL, et al. Effect of freeze-drying and gamma irradiation on the mechanical properties of human cancellous bone. J Orthop Res 2000;18:426–31.
50. Gazdag AR, Lane JM, Glaser D, et al. Alternatives to autogenous bone graft: efficacy and indications. J Am Acad Orthop Surg 1995;3:1–8.
51. Akkus O, Rimnac CM. Fracture resistance of gamma sterilized cortical bone allografts. J Orthop Res 2001;19:927–34.
52. Currey JD, Foreman J, Laketic I, et al. Effects of ionizing radiation on the mechanical properties of human bone. J Orthop Res 1997;15:111–7.
53. Akkus O, Belaney RM, Das P. Free radical scavenging alleviates the biomechanical impairment of gamma radiation sterilized bone tissue. J Orthop Res 2005;23(4):838–45.
54. Seto A, Gatt CJ Jr, Dunn MG. Radioprotection of tendon tissue via crosslinking and free radical scavenging. Clin Orthop Relat Res 2008; May 30.
55. Grieb TA, Forng RY, Stafford RE, et al. Effective use of optimized, high-dose (50 kGy) gamma irradiation for pathogen inactivation of human bone allografts. Biomaterials 2005;26(14):2033–42.
56. Grieb TA, Forng RY, Bogdansky S, et al. High-dose gamma irradiation for soft tissue allografts: high margin of safety with biomechanical integrity. J Orthop Res 2006;24(5):1011–8.
57. Rappe M, Horodyski M, Meister K, et al. Nonirradiated versus irradiated Achilles allograft: in vivo failure comparison. Am J Sports Med 2007;35(10):1653–8.
58. Schwartz HE, Matava MJ, Proch FS, et al. The effect of gamma irradiation on anterior cruciate ligament allograft biomechanical and biochemical properties in the caprine model at time zero and at 6 months after surgery. Am J Sports Med 2006;34(11):1747–55.
59. AATB. Standards for tissue banking. McLean (VA): American association of tissue banks; 2002.
60. Brockbank KG, Carpenter JF, Dawson PE. Effects of storage temperature on viable bioprosthetic heart valves. Cryobiology 1992;29:537–42.
61. Crawford MJ, Swenson CL, Arnoczky SP, et al. Lyophilization does not inactivate infectious retrovirus in systemically infected bone and tendon allografts. Am J Sports Med 2004;32:580–6.
62. Schimizzi A, Wedemeyer M, Odell T, et al. Effects of a novel sterilization process on soft tissue mechanical properties for anterior cruciate ligament allografts. Am J Sports Med 2007;35:612–6.

63. Jones DB, Huddleston PM, Zobitz ME, et al. Mechanical properties of patellar tendon allografts subjected to chemical sterilization. Arthroscopy 2007;23(4): 400–4.
64. Jordy A, Hoff-Jorgensen R, Flagstad A, et al. Virus inactivation by ethylene oxide containing gases. Acta Vet Scand 1975;16:379–87.
65. Prolo DJ, Pedrotti PW, White DH. Ethylene oxide sterilization of bone, dura mater, and fascia lata for human transplantation. Neurosurgery 1980;6:529–39.
66. Kakiuchi M, Ono K. Preparation of bank bone using defatting, freeze-drying and sterilisation with ethylene oxide gas. Part 2. Clinical evaluation of its efficacy and safety. Int Orthop 1996;20:147–52.
67. Kakiuchi M, Ono K, Nishimura A, et al. Preparation of bank bone using defatting, freeze-drying and sterilisation with ethylene oxide gas. Part 1. Experimental evaluation of its efficacy and safety. Int Orthop 1996;20:142–6.
68. Jackson DW, Windier GE, Simon TM. Intraarticular reaction associated with the use of freeze-dried, ethylene oxide-sterilized bone-patella tendon-bone allografts in the reconstruction of the anterior cruciate ligament. Am J Sports Med 1990;18: 1–11.
69. Roberts TS, Drez D Jr, McCarthy W, et al. Anterior cruciate ligament reconstruction using freeze-dried, ethylene oxidesterilized, bone-patellar tendon-bone allografts. Two year results in thirty-six patients. Am J Sports Med 1991;19:35–41.
70. Moore TM, Gendler E, Gendler E. Viruses adsorbed on musculoskeletal allografts are inactivated by terminal ethylene oxide disinfection. J Orthop Res 2004;22: 1358–61.
71. Campbell DG, Li P. Sterilization of HIV with irradiation: Relevance to infected bone allografts. Aust N Z J Surg 1999;69:517–21.
72. Conway B, Tomford W, Hirsch M, et al. Effects of gamma irradiation on HIV-1 in a bone allograft model. Trans Orthop Res Soc 1990;15:225.

Meniscus Replacement Using Synthetic Materials

Tony G. van Tienen, MD, PhD*, Gerjon Hannink, PhD, Pieter Buma, PhD

KEYWORDS

- Meniscus • Synthetic materials • Polymers
- Replacement • Repair

ANATOMY

The function of the meniscus is reflected in its anatomy because its cells and extracellular matrix are arranged in such a way that compressive forces, shear stresses, circumferentially directed forces, and tensile hoop stresses can be endured and redirected optimally.[1–3] During embryonic development, non-differentiated mesenchymal fibroblast-like progenitor cells differentiate into the highly specialized meniscus tissue. In general, the matrix of the meniscus is mainly composed of type I collagen, but a number of minor collagens (for instance types II, III, V, VI) and glycosaminoglycans (GAGs) are present in lower quantities, particularly associated with the fibrocartilaginous phenotype. The numerous collagen type I bundles, which are strong in tensile stress, are oriented in a circumferential direction and are considered to be very important in preventing radial extrusion of the meniscus and in maintaining the structural integrity of the meniscus during load bearing.[4,5] The GAGs play an important role in the maintenance of optimal visco-elastic behavior, compressive stiffness, and tissue hydration (78% is water). Furthermore, GAGs and surface zone proteins are thought to facilitate a smooth frictionless movement of the menisci over the articular surfaces of the tibia and femur.[4,5]

CONSEQUENCES OF MENISCUS RESECTION (PARTIAL VS. TOTAL, LOCATION OF TEAR)

Substantial damage to the meniscus can make a (subtotal) meniscectomy inevitable. In the 1960s and 1970s, a total meniscectomy was a common surgical intervention. The tear resulted in the locking phenomena and the abnormal stresses, which were the main causes of functional impairment and pain, and with the resection, the pain disappeared instantly. However, in time, it became clear that even a partial

Orthopedic Research Laboratory, Radboud University Nijmegen Medical Centre, P.O. Box 9101, 6500 HB, Nijmegen, The Netherlands
* Corresponding author.
E-mail address: t.vantienen@orthop.umcn.nl (T.G. van Tienen).

Clin Sports Med 28 (2009) 143–156
doi:10.1016/j.csm.2008.08.003
0278-5919/08/$ – see front matter © 2008 Elsevier Inc. All rights reserved.

sportsmed.theclinics.com

meniscectomy generates abnormal load stresses on articular cartilage, which lead to the development of osteoarthritic changes in tibia and femur.[6–8] Moreover, the damage to the cartilage appeared to be directly related to the amount of tissue removed.[6,9] Removal of (parts of) the lateral meniscus seemed to be more detrimental to the articular cartilage than removal of the medial meniscus. The fact that the lateral meniscus covers 76% of the articular cartilage instead of 60% on the medial side (partly) explains this difference.[10]

When more than 30% of the meniscus is removed during partial meniscectomy, preservation of the peripheral rim of the meniscus is essential to obtain the best long-term results,[11] probably because this remaining tissue is still able to transfer the axial joint load into hoop stresses and in this way restrict the peak stresses to the cartilage. The importance of the peripheral rim on the load transmission through the joint was earlier emphasized by Ahmed and colleagues.[10]

Tears in the posterior horn of the meniscus are common probably because of the increased transmitted load during the physiologic rollback of the femoral condyles with flexion of the knee joint. Experimental resection of the medial meniscus posterior horn in anterior cruciate ligament (ACL) intact cadaver knees has been demonstrated to have a significant effect on external rotational stability of the knee.[12] In purely anterior-posterior direction, this role is less.[13]

This diminished external rotation stability may play a role in the development of more articular cartilage damage after posterior horn resection, as shown in clinical studies.[11]

REPAIR

In view of the progressive osteoarthritic changes, a great deal of effort has been put into devices that fix the loose segment or a tear onto the main body of the meniscus, especially for the younger patient. Suturing is a safe traditional procedure but can be time-consuming. In addition, the rehabilitation after meniscectomy is usually quicker than after suturing, so the decision is often an ethical one, especially in the competitive athlete who wants to be back in training as soon as possible. However, when a meniscal tear occurs in combination with an ACL rupture, the results of meniscal suturing are relatively good, partly because the rehabilitation after ACL reconstruction offers the patient the time frame for an optimal healing period of the meniscus.[14]

Biomechanical tests under cyclic loading have shown that vertical sutures were superior to both horizontal sutures and knot-end techniques.[15] More recently, anchors, screws, staples, and a variety of other devices have been advocated for the rapid fixation of loose segments.[15,16] However, some of them might damage the articular cartilage when not completely sunk beneath the surface of the meniscus.[17]

The main problem in all repair techniques is that tears in the white zone of the meniscus, particularly in the slightly older patient, may only heal slowly or not at all because of insufficient blood vessel supply and a lack of recruitment of new cells. If tears do not heal, the mechanical forces might in time lead to failure of the fixation. Failure rates of menisci with sutured loose fragments of up to 28%[18] and 30%[19] have been reported in recent studies. However, in a recent overview article by Myers on the preservation of the meniscus, only a preliminary failure rate of 5.9% was reported.[14] A formal follow-up of these patients will be reported soon (PT Myers, personal communication, 2008).

In conclusion, one should always consider the possibility of repairing the meniscus, especially in the young active patient. The results of the repairs can be good when a proper technique is used and the patient is subjected to an adequate rehabilitation period. Especially in combination with a simultaneous ACL reconstruction, a repair seems to be attractive because the results are good and the rehabilitation could be integrated with that of the ACL reconstruction.

REPLACEMENT
Partial

When a partial menisectomy is performed and the peripheral meniscal rim is still intact, replacement of the resected tissue by a collagen scaffold (collagen meniscus implant [CMI]) might be an option. According to several studies, the importance of an intact peripheral rim cannot be emphasized enough. At this moment, the CMI is not approved by the FDA for sale in the United States and is currently the subject of a multi-center clinical trial. In Europe, the CMI is approved for use in a clinical setting for medial meniscus injury. The CMI is a collagen-based implant that acts as a temporary template for tissue infiltration and which in time seemed to have the ability to fill the defect with functional repair tissue and thereby may protect the articular cartilage from progressive osteoarthritis. These sponge-like scaffolds are made from bovine Achilles tendon-derived collagen and after addition of GAGs the structures are dehydrated, oriented in a mold, lyophilized, and chemically cross-linked with formaldehyde.[20] A number of clinical studies were published about the results of this CMI.[20–24] Most studies were performed by the original inventors of the CMI.[20–23] In the latest 2 prospective follow-up studies, 8 patients were followed for 5 to 6 years[22] and 6 to 8 years.[24] In the 5- to 6-year single-surgeon study, the medial meniscus was repaired. In general, the functional, activity, self-assessment, and pain scores improved significantly during the observation period. However, 2 patients had decreased Lysholm scores in the most recent follow-up and 4 had no changes. One patient mentioned increased pain at the latest follow-up evaluation but this was likely induced by a work-related injury. Imaging studies did not show progression of osteoarthritic changes of the medial compartment during the 5- to 8-year period. During the second-look arthroscopy, 69% of the original defect appeared to be filled with tissue, which was of a fibrocartilaginous nature (in 3 patients). No biomechanical test of the newly formed tissue was performed. Again, the investigators mention a large randomized trial of approximately 300 patients in which the CMI is compared with a partial meniscectomy. The first results of this study were presented at the European Society of Sports Traumatology, Knee Surgery and Arthroscopy-American Orthopaedic Society for Sports Medicine traveling meeting in Vail, Colorado. In this study, the original inventors of the CMI were not involved.[24] After 6 to 8 years follow-up, both the Cincinnati Knee Rating System (CKRS) and the International Knee Documentation Committee (IKDC) scores showed improvement in nearly all cases; however, magnetic resonance imaging (MRI) showed a myxoid degeneration signal in 5 cases, 2 had a normal signal with reduced size, while 1 patient had no recognizable implant. Six patients had preserved cartilage and articular space, with no changes with respect to the preoperative control. Interestingly, arthroscopic relook evaluation has been performed in 3 cases revealing the presence of the implant in 2 cases: 1 scaffold had shrunk, whereas in the other case, the CMI had almost disappeared.[24] At second-look arthroscopy, Choi and colleagues[25] took biopsies of the CMI-tissue construct in 128 patients 1 year after implantation. The tissue looked similar to native meniscus tissue. They still found some remnants of the CMI implant and in 8.6% of the cases, there was some synovitis in the joint. The collagen meniscus implant is biocompatible, resorbable, and may be easily remodeled by new infiltrating tissue. The main function of the CMI is to conduct tissue to differentiate into neo-meniscal tissue and thereby protect the articular cartilage. Indeed, tissue infiltration occurs in the CMI implant, and preclinical and clinical biopsies showed a differentiation into fibrocartilage-like tissue. However, synovitis was observed in several patients and so far, no biomechanical or chemical typing of the new extracellular matrix has been performed.

If the currently running prospective trial in the USA shows that the CMI is superior to partial meniscectomy in the prevention of further articular cartilage degradation, the market for the CMI may be large. According to the brochure of the manufacturing company, the first results seem to be positive: an increase in meniscal tissue after CMI implantation and an increase in Tegner activity level compared with the controls at 24 months.

Polyurethanes

Competition might be expected from polymers for the repair of partial resected tissue. As discussed later on, polyurothanes were initially developed and tested in animal studies for total meniscal replacement but are now being assessed as a scaffold for partial meniscal replacement as an alternative for the CMI.[26] The polyurethanes are believed to have better material properties to suture to the remaining tissue and to re-sist the extreme forces within the knee joint (**Fig. 1**). A prospective clinical trial, which is being performed at this moment, should reveal if this hypothesis would hold. The first preliminary results seem promising (**Fig. 2**). An animal study in partial replacement with similar material was presented by Brophy and colleagues.[27] They showed in sheep ca-davers that the contact pressures after partial meniscectomy and replacement with polyurethanes were less than the contact pressures after partial meniscectomy only.

Allograft (Donor Meniscus)

When patients have had a meniscectomy in the past and there is persistent pain on that ipsilateral side, meniscus allograft transplantation might be an option. Contraindi-cations are arthritis, because only Outerbridge grades 1 and 2 of cartilage damage are generally allowed for this procedure and an improper leg alignment. The latter can be corrected by an osteotomy. Although there is no upper age limit, the allograft

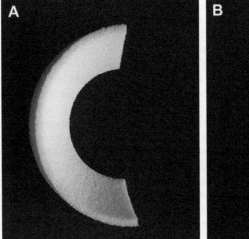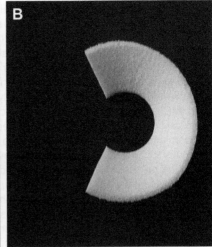

Fig. 1. Actifit porous polymers (*A*) for partial medial menisectomy, (*B*) for lateral menisectomy. (*Courtesy of* Orteq Bioengineering, London, UK; with permission.)

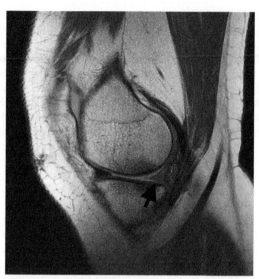

Fig. 2. MRI scan, which shows the medial meniscus 3 mo after resection of the posterior horn and implantation of the polycaprolacton polyurethane implant (Actifit) (*arrow*). (*Courtesy of* Peter Verdonk and Orteq Bioengeneering, London, UK; with permission.)

replacement procedure is generally performed in patients below the age of 50 years.[28] There is still controversy about the painful knee after a *recent* meniscectomy. However, general opinion remains to postpone the procedure with careful follow-up using regular X-rays or MRI to choose the right timing.

Disappointing results are often associated with too severe osteoarthritis,[29] improper leg alignment,[30–32] and irradiated donor menisci.[33] By addressing all those requirements, reported success rates are between 60% and 94%.[29–32,34–40] Also, a very recent study by Wills and Laprade showed excellent results 2 years after allograft transplantation.[41]

However, worldwide the amounts of these replacements remain low not only because of the varying results but also the availability, difficult logistics, and costs of the transplant. Recently, an article was published on the decellularization process of porcine meniscus.[42] This xenograft could then be used as a scaffold for tissue regeneration after implantation in humans. The remaining tissue after processing seemed to be of good biomechanical quality and not cytotoxic in cell culture. This may be an alternative for allografts in the future. Nevertheless, the search for an artificial replacement material is still going on.

PRESENT STATUS

Although the literature addresses merely the *total* replacement of the meniscus in animal studies, the current clinical studies only concern *partial* replacement (CMI) of the resected meniscus. To the authors' knowledge, no clinical studies have been published in which the entire meniscus was replaced by an artificial material. The first animal studies on meniscus replacement go back to the early 1980s, and in the following years, there was further development of porous (tissue-conductive) materials. In 1983, the first publication suggested the use of a histocompatible Teflon net for ingrowth of regenerating meniscal tissue.[43] Although the authors commented on the regenerative effect of the material and the function of the knee joint as hopeful, later studies on this material were never reported. Messner and colleagues[44,45] started to use polyurethane-coated Teflon or Dacron for meniscal replacement in rabbits and published these results in 1992.[46] The coating seemed favorable for infiltration of tissue; however, all the joints showed signs of degeneration and osteoarthritis. In addition, coverage of the implant with periosteal tissue did not lead to favorable results.[47] Simultaneously, the authors' group started collaboration between a polymer chemistry department and an orthopedic research laboratory to develop a biodegradable porous polymer as a scaffold for meniscal tissue regeneration. They hypothesized that a porous scaffold could have a tissue conductive function to guide the infiltrating multi-potent tissue from the synovium into the joint. In 1944, Smillie reported some regenerative capacity in humans; however, it is now known that this capacity is limited.[48] Experimental studies from Moon showed the regenerating capacity in animals.[49] Based on this regenerative capacity, an attempt was made to develop a temporary scaffold that allowed tissue infiltration and matrix formation, that is, collagen and GAGs, and later the scaffold was presumed to degrade in nontoxic particles. The first scaffolds consisted of polyurethanes reinforced with carbon fibers.[50] However, the carbon particles induced a synovial inflammation causing extra damage to the joint. Nevertheless, tissue infiltration proved to be possible with porous materials. Newer materials with polyurethanes as the basis proved to be superior: they were used for meniscus replacement in dogs, and after 6 to 12 weeks, the scaffold was filled with tissue and even had some cartilage protective effect on macroscopic evaluation.[51] The amount of fibrocartilage formation in these scaffolds seemed to be influenced by the initial stiffness of the scaffold: the closer the stiffness approached that of the native meniscus stiffness the more fibrocartilage was formed. The challenge was to produce an open structure scaffold (for tissue infiltration) that is still stiff enough to enable fibrocartilage formation. The authors succeeded in developing a polyurethane-based polycaprolactone scaffold with a high stiffness and an adequate amount of pores and replaced the lateral meniscus in beagle dogs.[52] After 6 months, tissue infiltration and fibrocartilage formation were observed in the polymers; however, a disappointing amount of cartilage damage was found: the implantation did not prevent articular cartilage damage, the initial goal of the studies. Also, on the longer term (2 years follow-up), the scaffold initially filled with fibrocartilage-like tissue but later on the core of the scaffolds became acellular with the extracellular matrix still in place. The decrease in amount of blood vessels in time may have been an explanation. In contrast, the implants did not cause any severe synovitis and microscopically there were no distinct signs of foreign body reaction from the degradation products. Considering the results at this stage, this research seems not to justify replacement of the *whole* meniscus with this polymer in a clinical setting. As discussed earlier in this article, partial replacement of resected meniscus with this new material might be a valuable alternative at this stage (see paragraph "Partial replacement").

Recently, several experimental articles have been published on artificial meniscus replacement. A research group from Bologna, Italy, reported the effects of replacement of the meniscus with a material based on polycaprolactone and hyaluronic acid (PCL/HYAFF). This experiment is part of a research line supported by the European Commission Fifth Framework Program (Project title: Innovative materials and technologies for a bio-engineered meniscus substitute, Project No. GRD1-2001-40,401, Contract No G5RD-CT).[53] In a sheep model, they succeeded in producing a porous scaffold that enabled vascularized tissue infiltration 6 weeks after surgery. However, it seemed hard to protect the knee from arthritis and the implant tended to be extruded from the joint to some extent. Longer-term follow-up studies with this scaffold show very promising results and are yet to be published (personal communication) (**Figs. 3** and **4**). This study

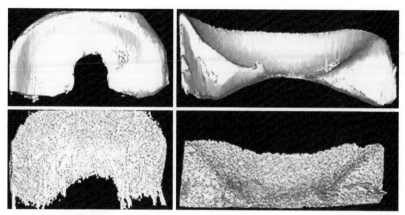

Fig. 3. PCL-HYAFF porous medial meniscus scaffold. (*Courtesy of* E. Kon and M. Delcogliano, Rizolli Orthopedic Institute Bologna; with permission.)

also showed that seeding of the scaffolds with autologous chondrocytes provides some benefit in the extent of fibrocartilaginous tissue repair. A Japanese study used a polyvinyl-alcohol hydrogel scaffold in rabbits. This study seemed to be more successful in terms of cartilage degeneration (less than in the meniscectomy group).[54] However, the material properties needed to be improved to provide higher tear strength for suturing it to the synovium. Other material features such as stiffness and wear- or degradation characteristics were not provided. No later reports were published by this group on this subject.

There are also some publications about meniscal cell regeneration in vitro (**Table 1**). Especially the group of Athanasiou remains active in this field. Recently, they suggested the use of Agar gels for meniscal cell growth in vitro with favorable results.[55] The biomechanical and histologic features seemed to resemble the native meniscus tissue. A Japanese study showed the increased regenerative and reparative effect on meniscal cells when added on a platelet-rich plasma gel.[56]

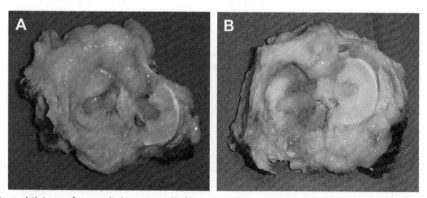

Fig. 4. (*A*) 4 mo after medial meniscus (*left*) replacement, cell-seeded implants, (*B*) non-seeded implants (*left*). (*Courtesy of* E. Kon and M. Delcogliano, Rizolli Orthopedic Institute Bologna; with permission.)

Table 1
Experimental scaffold materials (and cell-seeding techniques) for meniscal replacement

Scaffold Structure (Experimental)	In Vivo/Vitro Study	Conclusions
Polycaprolacton polyurethanes		
Polycaprolacton[62] foam scaffold	In vivo dog study follow-up 6 mo	Almost identical compression behavior as native meniscus. No significant differences in collagen I or II and PG compared with native meniscus
Polycaprolacton[63] (not) aligned nanofibers	In vitro stem cell seeding on scaffolds. follow-up 70 d.	All nanofibrous scaffolds serve as a micro-pattern for directed tissue growth and, when seeded with stem cells, produce constructs with improved mechanical properties compared with non-seeded scaffolds.
Polycaprolacton[26,50] foam scaffold	In vivo follow-up 6 mo in dogs	Fibrovascular tissue infiltration. Collagen II and proteoglycans production. However, articular damage could not be prevented.
Polycaprolacton and hyaluronic acid foam (HYAFF 11).[58,64] Specific orientation of the pores in the structure	In vitro MSC follow-up 6 days And In vivo sheep follow-up 6 wk	MSCs grown on the scaffold expressed collagen type I, type III, fibronectin, laminin, and actin. Well attached to capsule, tissue infiltration in scaffold; however, cartilage damage could not be prevented.
Polyglycolic acid		
Hydrogel agarose versus non-woven GA mesh[55]	In vitro chondrocyte (AC)/ meniscal fibrochondrocyte (MFC) mix cultures on agarose and PGA mesh follow-up 8 wk	High-density cell cocultures of ACs and MFCs (without scaffold) resulted in stiffer constructs, higher tensile modulus, and more collagen type 1 than cells seeded on PGA mesh.
Polyglycolic acid mesh.[65] Nonbonded or bonded with PGLactic acid to reinforce scaffold	In vitro follow up 1 wk with meniscal chondrocytes, In vivo follow-up 10 and 36 wk rabbits	Non-seeded scaffolds deformed after 10 wk implantation. 36 wk: Cell-seeded scaffolds: more total collagen in middle region but less total collagen in outer region (horns) than native meniscus, less tibial articular cartilage damage than that with non–cell-seeded scaffolds

Other materials		
Polyvinyl-alcohol-hyaluronic acid mesh[54]	In vivo follow-up 2 y implanted in rabbits	No progression of OA after 1 year of implantation compared with menisectomy. After 2 years, no breakage or displacement of implant was observed. Stress–strain curves did not differ from normal menisci
Carbon-fiber reinforced polyurethane-polylactic acid mesh[54,66]	In vivo follow-up 19 wk dogs	Ingrowth of fibrous/fibrocartilaginous tissue and vessels. Synovitis.

FUTURE

The meniscus appears to be a sophisticated piece of tissue able to withstand the huge forces inside the knee joint. It has the ideal strength, gliding, and shock absorbing capacity to reduce peak stresses in the knee joint. Until now, the properties of this tissue seemed hard to mimic and the underlying cartilage seemed very vulnerable. While earlier studies looked more into a permanent "nonbiological" solution, recent studies focused on (degrading) porous tissue-conductive scaffolds. The latter option endeavors a living and non-wearing substitute for the meniscus and, therefore, many material requirements need to be addressed:

- The material needs to be open to enable the tissue to grow in (high porosity).
- To withstand the initial forces (before the tissue grows in), it needs to be as stiff and strong as the native meniscus.
- To mimic the tribology of the native meniscus.
- To hold the sutures it also needs to be tear resistant.
- If degradable, then timing of the degradation is essential (not before the tissue has grown in).
- If degradable, then its products need to be nontoxic.
- The material and its degradation products may not evoke a foreign body reaction.

REALIZATION

With the presently available salt leaching techniques, the authors and other groups were able to create open structures in polymers with acceptable biomechanical properties.[57,58] Recently, techniques such as rapid prototyping have been developed to fabricate three-dimensional scaffolds for tissue-engineering purposes. The mechanical properties of many different soft and hard tissues, including bovine cartilage, could be mimicked by these copolymers by using a three-dimensional fiber deposition technique, simply by varying the scaffold porosity, the scaffold architecture, and/or the copolymer composition.[59]

   With these techniques, it may be possible to guide the infiltrating tissue into the preferable direction, for example, peripheral collagen fibers into peripheral circumferential tunnels, to better withstand hoop stresses during loading of the joint. Furthermore, these techniques may improve the biomechanical properties of the scaffolds and, as such, their initial performance in the knee joint before the actual tissue infiltration is completed. Subsequently, initial articular cartilage damage might be decreased

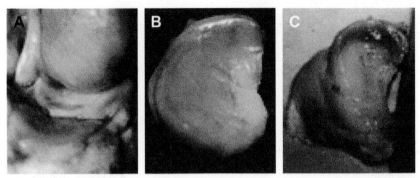

Fig. 5. Appearance of regenerated medial meniscus after intra-articular treatment with autologous MSCs. The cell treatment resulted in the formation of tissue in the posterior compartment 12 wk after complete medial meniscectomy. The excised tissues (*B* and *C*) inserted between the distal head of the femur and proximal tibial plateau (*A*) are shown. (*From* Murphy JM, Fink DJ, Hunziker EB, et al. Stem cell therapy in a caprine model of osteoarthritis. Arthritis & Rheumatism 2003;48(12):3464–74; with permission. © 2003, American College of Rheumatology. Reprinted with permission of Wiley-Liss, Inc., a subsidiary of John Wiley & Sons, Inc.)

as seen in the authors' studies.[50] Also in terms of sizing the scaffold, these techniques may be a valuable addition. From experiences in allograft meniscal transplantation, the relevance of the proper implant size is fully recognized.[60]

With stem cell therapy a new era was entered and may also be a promising option for cartilage and meniscus regeneration. Murphy and Barry published an impressive study on this technique in goats.[61] They injected mesenchymal stem cells (MSCs) in osteoarthritic knees as a result of earlier ACL transection and lateral menisectomy. Pictures show meniscus-like regenerative tissue with collagen type II present as a sign of hyaline matrix formation (**Fig. 5**). The MSCs were part of the repair tissue. Together with in vitro tissue engineering as summarized in **Table 1**, stem cell therapy may play an important role in getting closer to the solution of eventual total replacement of the meniscus in a clinical setting.

With increasing awareness that a total menisectomy leads to severe arthritis, the indication for a total meniscus replacement may be less in time. Consequently, the amount of partial menisectomies may even increase and, subsequently, the need for partial replacement techniques. Hence, in the development of an artificial meniscus, it would be very advantageous if this material can also be employed to replace only the resected tissue. This makes the material more widely applicable. At this moment, 2 different materials are subject to clinical trials. As stated before, these studies only include patients with partial menisectomies, and only the resected tissue is replaced with these materials. Until now, the only available clinical option for total meniscus replacement is the use of allograft meniscus. The material requirements for artificial *total* meniscus replacement are not fully addressed yet, that is, cartilage damage has not yet been prevented.

REFERENCES

1. DeHaven KE. The role of the meniscus. In: Ewing JW, editor. Articular cartilage and knee joint function: basic science and arthroscopy. New York (NY): Raven Press, Ltd.; 1990. p. 103–15.

2. Fithian DC, Kelly MA, Mow VC. Material properties and structure-function relationships in the menisci. Clin Orthop Relat Res 1990;(252):19–31.
3. Walker PS, Erkman MJ. The role of the menisci in force transmission across the knee. Clin Orthop Relat Res 1975;(109):184–92.
4. Ghosh P, Taylor TK. The knee joint meniscus. A fibrocartilage of some distinction. Clin Orthop Relat Res 1987;(224):52–63.
5. Setton LA, Guilak F, Hsu EW, et al. Biomechanical factors in tissue engineered meniscal repair. Clin Orthop Relat Res 1999;(367 Suppl):254–72.
6. Cox JS, Nye CE, Schaefer WW, et al. The degenerative effects of partial and total resection of the medial meniscus in dogs' knees. Clin Orthop Relat Res 1975;(109):178–83.
7. Jaureguito JW, Elliot JS, Lietner T, et al. The effects of arthroscopic partial lateral meniscectomy in an otherwise normal knee: a retrospective review of functional, clinical, and radiographic results. Arthroscopy 1995;11:29–36.
8. Maletius W, Messner K. The effect of partial meniscectomy on the long-term prognosis of knees with localized, severe chondral damage. A twelve- to fifteen-year followup. Am J Sports Med 1996;24:258–62.
9. Englund M, Lohmander LS. Risk factors for symptomatic knee osteoarthritis fifteen to twenty-two years after meniscectomy. Arthritis Rheum 2004;50:2811–9.
10. Ahmed AM. The load-bearing role of the knee meniscus. In: Mow VC, Arnoczky SP, Jackson DW, editors. Knee meniscus: basic and clinical foundations. New York (NY): Raven Press, Ltd.; 1992. p. 59–73.
11. Hede A, Larsen E, Sandberg H. The long term outcome of open total and partial meniscectomy related to the quantity and site of the meniscus removed. Int Orthop 1992;16:122–5.
12. Watanabe Y, Scyoc AV, Tsuda E, et al. Biomechanical function of the posterior horn of the medial meniscus: a human cadaveric study. J Orthop Sci 2004;9:280–4.
13. Levy IM, Torzilli PA, Fish ID. The contribution of the menisci to the stability of the knee. In: Mow VC, Arnoczky SP, Jackson DW, editors. Knee meniscus: basic and clinical foundations. New York: Raven Press, Ltd.; 1992. p. 107–15.
14. Boyd KT, Myers PT. Meniscus preservation; rationale, repair techniques and results. Knee 2003;10:1–11.
15. Farng E, Sherman O. Meniscal repair devices: a clinical and biomechanical literature review. Arthroscopy 2004;20:273–86.
16. Miller MD, Kline AJ, Jepsen KG. "All-inside" meniscal repair devices: an experimental study in the goat model. Am J Sports Med 2004;32:858–62.
17. Laprell H, Stein V, Petersen W. Arthroscopic all-inside meniscus repair using a new refixation device: a prospective study. Arthroscopy 2002;18:387–93.
18. Kurzweil PR, Friedman MJ. Meniscus: resection, repair, and replacement. Arthroscopy 2002;18:33–9.
19. Lee GP, Diduch DR. Deteriorating outcomes after meniscal repair using the Meniscus Arrow in knees undergoing concurrent anterior cruciate ligament reconstruction: increased failure rate with long-term follow-up. Am J Sports Med 2005;33:1138–41.
20. Rodkey WG, Steadman JR, Li ST. A clinical study of collagen meniscus implants to restore the injured meniscus. Clin Orthop Relat Res 1999;367(Suppl):281–92.
21. Reguzzoni M, Manelli A, Ronga M, et al. Histology and ultrastructure of a tissue-engineered collagen meniscus before and after implantation. J Biomed Mater Res B Appl Biomater 2005;74:808–16.
22. Steadman JR, Rodkey WG. Tissue-engineered collagen meniscus implants: 5- to 6-year feasibility study results. Arthroscopy 2005;21:515–25.

23. Stone KR, Steadman JR, Rodkey WG, et al. Regeneration of meniscal cartilage with use of a collagen scaffold. Analysis of preliminary data. J Bone Joint Surg Am 1997;79:1770–7.
24. Zaffagnini S, Giordano G, Vascellari A, et al. Arthroscopic collagen meniscus implant results at 6 to 8 years follow up. Knee Surg Sports Traumatol Arthrosc 2007; 15:175–83.
25. Choi G, Vigorita VJ, DiCarlo EF. Second-look biopsy study of human collagen meniscal implants: A histological analysis of 81 cases [abstract 128]. In: Proceedings of the 75th Annual Meeting of the AAOS. San Francisco: American Academy of Orthopaedic Surgeons; 2008.
26. Tienen TG, Heijkants RG, Buma P, et al. A porous polymer scaffold for meniscal lesion repair–a study in dogs. Biomaterials 2003;24:2541–8.
27. Brophy R, Cottrell J, Deng XH, et al. Dynamic contact mechanics of a scaffold for partial meniscal replacement [abstract 125]. In: Proceedings of the 75th Annual Meeting of the AAOS. San Francisco: American Academy of Orthopaedic Surgeons; 2008.
28. Cole BJ, Carter TR, Rodeo SA. Allograft meniscal transplantation: background, techniques, and results. Instr Course Lect 2003;52:383–96.
29. Noyes FR, Barber-Westin SD. Irradiated meniscus allografts in the human knee. A two to five year follow-up study. Orthop Trans 1995;19:417.
30. van Arkel ER, de Boer HH. Survival analysis of human meniscal transplantations. J Bone Joint Surg Br 2002;84:227–31.
31. van Arkel ER, Goei R, de Pl, et al. Meniscal allografts: evaluation with magnetic resonance imaging and correlation with arthroscopy. Arthroscopy 2000;16:517–21.
32. van Arkel ER, de Boer HH. Human meniscal transplantation. Preliminary results at 2 to 5-year follow-up. J Bone Joint Surg Br 1995;77:589–95.
33. Yahia LH, Drouin G, Zukor D. The irradiation effect on the initial mechanical properties of meniscal grafts. Biomed Mater Eng 1993;3:211–21.
34. Milachowski KA, Weismeier K, Wirth CJ. Homologous meniscus transplantation. Experimental and clinical results. Int Orthop 1989;13:1–11.
35. Garret JC. Free meniscal transplantation: a prospective study of 44 cases. Arthroscopy 1993;9:368–9.
36. Cameron HU, Macnab I. The structure of the meniscus of the human knee joint. Clin Orthop Relat Res 1972;89:215–9.
37. Cameron JC, Saha S. Meniscal allograft transplantation for unicompartmental arthritis of the knee. Clin Orthop Relat Res 1997;337:164–71.
38. Goble EM, Kohn D, Verdonk R, et al. Meniscal substitutes–human experience. Scand J Med Sci Sports 1999;9:146–57.
39. Rath E, Richmond JC, Yassir W, et al. Meniscal allograft transplantation. Two- to eight-year results. Am J Sports Med 2001;29:410–4.
40. Rath E, Richmond JC. The menisci: basic science and advances in treatment. Br J Sports Med 2000;34:252–7.
41. Wills NJ, LaPrade RF. Clinical outcomes of meniscal allografts [abstract 127]. In: Proceedings of the 75th Annual Meeting of the AAOS. San Francisco: American Academy of Orthopaedic Surgeons; 2008.
42. Stapleton TW, Ingram J, Katta J, et al. Development and characterization of an acellular porcine medial meniscus for use in tissue engineering. Tissue Eng Part A 2008;14:505–18.
43. Toyonaga T, Uezaki N, Chikama H. Substitute meniscus of Teflon-net for the knee joint of dogs. Clin Orthop Relat Res 1983;179:291–7.

44. Messner K, Gillquist J. Prosthetic replacement of the rabbit medial meniscus. J Biomed Mater Res 1993;27:1165–73.
45. Messner K, Fahlgren A, Persliden J, et al. Radiographic joint space narrowing and histologic changes in a rabbit meniscectomy model of early knee osteoarthrosis. Am J Sports Med 2001;29:151–60.
46. Sommerlath K, Gillquist J. The effect of a meniscal prosthesis on knee biomechanics and cartilage. An experimental study in rabbits. Am J Sports Med 1992;20:73–81.
47. Messner K, Lohmander LS, Gillquist J. Cartilage mechanics and morphology, synovitis and proteoglycan fragments in rabbit joint fluid after prosthetic meniscal substitution. Biomaterials 1993;14:163–8.
48. Smillie IS. Observation on the regeneration of the semilunar cartilage in man. Br J Surg 1944;31:398–401.
49. Moon MS, Kim JM, Ok IY. The normal and regenerated meniscus in rabbits. Morphologic and histologic studies. Clin Orthop Relat Res 1984;182:264–9.
50. Tienen TG, Heijkants RG, de Groot JH, et al. Replacement of the knee meniscus by a porous polymer implant: a study in dogs. Am J Sports Med 2006;34:64–71.
51. Klompmaker J, Veth RP, Jansen HW, et al. Meniscal replacement using a porous polymer prosthesis: a preliminary study in the dog. Biomaterials 1996;17:1169–75.
52. Tienen TG, Heijkants RG, de Groot JH, et al. Meniscal replacement in dogs. Tissue regeneration in two different materials with similar properties. J Biomed Mater Res B Appl Biomater 2006;76:389–96.
53. Marsano A, Wendt D, Quinn TM, et al. Bi-zonal cartilaginous tissues engineered in a rotary cell culture system. Biorheology 2006;43:553–60.
54. Kobayashi M, Chang YS, Oka M. A two year in vivo study of polyvinyl alcohol-hydrogel (PVA-H) artificial meniscus. Biomaterials 2005;26:3243–8.
55. Aufderheide AC, Athanasiou KA. Assessment of a bovine co-culture, scaffold-free method for growing meniscus-shaped constructs. Tissue Eng 2007;13:2195–205.
56. Ishida K, Kuroda R, Miwa M, et al. The regenerative effects of platelet-rich plasma on meniscal cells in vitro and its in vivo application with biodegradable gelatin hydrogel. Tissue Eng 2007;13:1103–12.
57. de Groot JH, Zijlstra FM, Kuipers HW, et al. Meniscal tissue regeneration in porous 50/50 copoly(L-lactide/epsilon-caprolactone) implants. Biomaterials 1997;18:613–22.
58. Chiari C, Koller U, Dorotka R, et al. A tissue engineering approach to meniscus regeneration in a sheep model. Osteoarthritis Cartilage 2006;14:1056–65.
59. Moroni L, Poort G, Van KF, et al. Dynamic mechanical properties of 3D fiber-deposited PEOT/PBT scaffolds: an experimental and numerical analysis. J Biomed Mater Res A 2006;78:605–14.
60. Dienst M, Greis PE, Ellis BJ, et al. Effect of lateral meniscal allograft sizing on contact mechanics of the lateral tibial plateau: an experimental study in human cadaveric knee joints. Am J Sports Med 2007;35:34–42.
61. Murphy JM, Fink DJ, Hunziker EB, et al. Stem cell therapy in a caprine model of osteoarthritis. Arthritis Rheum 2003;48:3464–74.
62. Heijkants RG, van Calck RV, de Groot JH, et al. Design, synthesis and properties of a degradable polyurethane scaffold for meniscus regeneration. J Mater Sci Mater Med 2004;15:423–7.

63. Baker BM, Mauck RL. The effect of nanofiber alignment on the maturation of engineered meniscus constructs. Biomaterials 2007;28:1967–77.
64. Cristino S, Grassi F, Toneguzzi S, et al. Analysis of mesenchymal stem cells grown on a three-dimensional HYAFF 11-based prototype ligament scaffold. J Biomed Mater Res A 2005;73:275–83.
65. Kang SW, Son SM, Lee JS, et al. Regeneration of whole meniscus using meniscal cells and polymer scaffolds in a rabbit total meniscectomy model. J Biomed Mater Res A 2006;78:659–71.
66. Veth RP, Jansen HW, Leenslag JW, et al. Experimental meniscal lesions reconstructed with a carbon fiber-polyurethane-poly(L-lactide) graft. Clin Orthop Relat Res 1986;286–93.

Orthopedic Interface Tissue Engineering for the Biological Fixation of Soft Tissue Grafts

Kristen L. Moffat, MS[a], I-Ning Elaine Wang, MS[a], Scott A. Rodeo, MD[b], Helen H. Lu, PhD[a],*

KEYWORDS

- Interface tissue engineering • Enthesis
- Anterior cruciate ligament • Rotator cuff
- Scaffold • Co-culture • Tri-culture

A significant challenge in orthopedic reconstruction surgery resides in achieving extended functional integration of soft tissue grafts with subchondral bone. The biological fixation of these grafts is particularly critical in the repair of injuries to ligaments and tendons, because integration between soft and hard tissues is essential for musculoskeletal motion. Many soft tissues, such as the anterior cruciate ligament (ACL) or the supraspinatus tendon, exhibit direct insertions into subchondral bone through a complex enthesis consisting of 3 distinct yet continuous regions of soft tissue, fibrocartilage, and bone.[1–3] The fibrocartilage region is further divided into calcified and uncalcified zones. This multi-tissue organization serves several purposes, from mediating load transfer between ligament and bone[2,4] to minimizing the formation of stress concentrations[2,5,6] and to supporting the heterotypic cellular communication necessary for interface function and homeostasis.[7] The insertion site is, however, prone to injury, and mechanical fixation of current ligament or tendon reconstruction grafts often fail to preserve or reestablish an anatomic soft tissue-to-bone enthesis post-surgery. Absence of this critical interface has been reported to compromise graft stability and long-term clinical outcome.[8–11] Consequently, there exists a significant need for integrative graft fixation systems, which can promote interface regeneration and facilitate functional graft-to-bone integration.

[a] Department of Biomedical Engineering, Biomaterials and Interface Tissue Engineering Laboratory, Columbia University, 1210 Amsterdam Avenue, 351 Engineering Terrace Building, MC 8904, New York, NY 10027, USA
[b] The Hospital for Special Surgery, 535 East 70th Street, New York, NY 10021, USA
* Corresponding author.
E mail address: hl2052@columbia.edu (H.H. Lu).

Clin Sports Med 28 (2009) 157–176
doi:10.1016/j.csm.2008.08.006
0278-5919/08/$ – see front matter © 2008 Elsevier Inc. All rights reserved.

sportsmed.theclinics.com

In the past decade, tissue engineering[12,13] has emerged as a promising approach to musculoskeletal tissue repair and regeneration. Using a combination of cells, growth factors, and/or biomaterials, tremendous advances have been made, whereby bone-,[14–18] cartilage-,[19–23] tendon-,[24–28] and ligament-like[29–34] tissues have been engineered in vitro and in vivo. Design methodologies developed from these efforts can be readily applied to regenerate the enthesis between soft tissue and bone through interface tissue engineering. Focusing on the anterior cruciate ligament (ACL)-to-bone insertion site, this review highlights recent work in interface tissue engineering, aimed at promoting the biological fixation of grafts used for ACL reconstruction surgery. Current knowledge of the mechanism of interface regeneration, elucidation of the structure and function relationship inherent at the ligament-to-bone insertion, and implementation of strategic biomimicry in stratified scaffold design for interface regeneration are discussed. Extension of these interface tissue engineering strategies to rotator cuff repair is also highlighted. Finally, potential challenges and future directions in this emerging field are considered. It is emphasized that biological fixation through interface tissue engineering will be instrumental in the development of a new generation of *integrative* fixation devices and the design of complex musculoskeletal tissue systems that can integrate seamlessly with the body.

DESIGN CONSIDERATIONS IN ACL–BONE INTERFACE TISSUE ENGINEERING

Ligaments or tendons insert into bone through either direct or indirect entheses, with the latter characterized by soft tissue attachment to the periosteum and Sharpey's fibers traversing directly from the soft tissue to bone.[4] In contrast, direct insertions, exhibited by the ACL or supraspinatus tendon, are much more complex, transiting from soft tissue to bone through a characteristic fibrocartilage interface, which is further divided into non-mineralized and mineralized regions.[1–3,35–41] The ACL-to-bone junction exhibits controlled spatial variations in cell type and matrix composition (**Fig. 1**), with the ligament proper composed of fibroblasts embedded in a type I and type III collagen matrix. The non-mineralized fibrocartilage matrix consists of ovoid chondrocytes, and types I and II collagen are present within a proteoglycan-rich matrix. In the mineralized fibrocartilage zone, hypertrophic chondrocytes are surrounded by a calcified matrix containing type X collagen.[40,42] The last region is the subchondral bone, within which osteoblasts, osteocytes, and osteoclasts reside in a mineralized type I collagen matrix. This controlled matrix heterogeneity observed at the interface reduces the accumulation of stress concentrations and facilitates the transfer of complex loads between soft and hard tissues.[2,6,43]

The ACL is also the most frequently injured knee ligament,[44] with 200,000 injuries and approximately 100,000 reconstruction procedures reported annually in the United States alone.[45,46] The long-term performance of ACL grafts depends on the structural and material properties of the graft, initial graft tension,[47–51] the intra-articular position of the graft,[52,53] and graft fixation.[9,10] Increased emphasis has been placed on graft fixation because post-surgical rehabilitation regimens require the immediate ability to regain the full range of motion, re-establish neuromuscular function, and bear weight.[11,54] Autologous hamstring or allografts are increasingly used for ACL reconstruction due to donor site morbidity associated with bone-patellar tendon-bone grafts (BPTB).[55,56] The BPTB graft has been the gold standard, in part because of its ability to integrate with subchondral bone through its bony ends. Moreover, it possesses intact insertion sites or entheses that can serve as functional transitions between soft tissue and bone. In contrast, the tendinous grafts must be fixed mechanically within the bone tunnel. Although the physiologic range of motion may be possible by way of mechanical fixation, graft-to-bone integration is not achieved

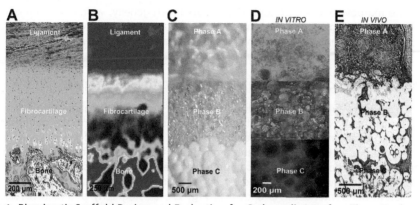

Fig. 1. Biomimetic Scaffold Design and Evaluation for Orthopedic Interface Tissue Engineering. (*A*) The native ACL-bone interface exhibits distinct yet continuous tissue regions, including ligament, fibrocartilage, and bone. (Neonatal Bovine, Modified Goldner Masson Trichrome Stain, bar = 200 μm). (*B*) Fourier Transform Infrared Spectroscopic Imaging (FTIR-I) revealed that relative collagen content is the highest in the ligament and bone regions, with a decrease in collagen across the fibrocartilage interface from ligament to bone (neonatal bovine, bar = 250 μm, with *blue* to *red* representing low to high collagen content, respectively). (*C*) A tri-phasic stratified scaffold has been designed to mimic the 3 distinct yet continuous interface regions (bar = 500 μm). (*D*) *In vitro* co-culture of fibroblasts and osteoblasts on the tri-phasic scaffold resulted in phase-specific cell distribution and cell-specific matrix deposition. Fibroblasts (Calcein AM, *green*) were localized in Phase A and osteoblasts (CM-Dil, *red*) in Phase C over time. Both osteoblasts and fibroblasts migrated into Phase B by d 28 (bar = 200 μm). (*E*) *In vivo* evaluation of the tri-phasic scaffold tri-cultured with fibroblasts (Phase A), chondrocytes (Phase B), and osteoblasts (Phase C) revealed abundant host tissue infiltration and matrix production (wk 4, Modified Goldner Masson Trichrome Stain, bar = 500 μm).

because the native insertion site is lost during surgery, with non-mineralized soft tissue found instead within the bone tunnels.[9,11,57] Thus graft fixation at the tibial and femoral tunnels, instead of the isolated strength of the graft, represent the weakest point during the early postoperative healing period.[9,10,58] Despite improvement in fixation with interference screws, the clinical outcomes of ACL reconstructions with hamstring tendon grafts have continued to be afflicted with greater laxity and higher failure rates compared with BPTB reconstructions.[59–66] In the absence of an anatomic interface, the graft-bone junction exhibits poor mechanical stability,[9,10,58] which remains one of the primary causes of graft failure.[8–10,67,68]

Based on the intricate multi-tissue organization observed at the soft tissue-to-bone junction, it is likely that interface formation will require *multiple types* of cells, a *multiphased* scaffold system that supports interactions between these different cell populations, and the development of distinct yet continuous *multi-tissue regions* mimicking that of the native insertion through physical and biochemical stimuli. Moreover, the success of any interface tissue engineering effort first requires an in-depth understanding of the structure–function relationship at the native insertion to identify interface-relevant design parameters. In addition, the mechanism governing interface regeneration must be determined, especially the role of heterotypic cellular interactions in interface repair and homeostasis. Multi-scale co-culture or tri-culture models may be used to decipher the relative contribution of homotypic and heterotypic cellular communication in multi-tissue regeneration. This knowledge will enable the design of stratified scaffolds optimized for supporting heterotypic cellular interactions and promote the development of controlled matrix heterogeneity, which is essential for interface tissue engineering. Recent advances in each of the above 3 critical areas in interface tissue engineering are highlighted in the following sections.

STRUCTURE–FUNCTION RELATIONSHIP AT THE LIGAMENT-TO-BONE INTERFACE

From a structure–function perspective, the complex multi-tissue organization and heterogeneity in matrix composition at the interface are likely related to the nature and distribution of the mechanical stress experienced at the ligament–bone junction. It has been reported that matrix organization at soft tissue-to-bone transitions is optimized to sustain both tensile and compressive stresses.[4,69,70] Recently, using ultrasound elastography,[71] Spalazzi and colleagues[72] mapped the strain distribution at the ACL-to-bone interface. As shown in **Fig. 2**A, elastography analyses revealed that when the joint is loaded in tension, the deformation across the insertion site is region-dependent, with the highest displacement observed at the ACL, followed by a decrease from the fibrocartilage interface to bone. These regional differences suggest an increase in tissue stiffness from ligament to bone. In addition, both tensile and

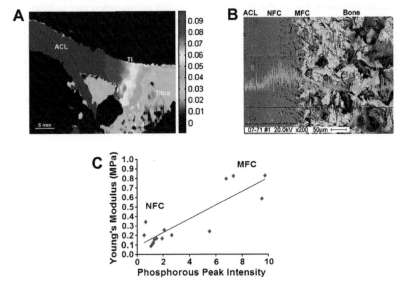

Fig. 2. Structure–Function Relationship at the Ligament-to-Bone Insertion Site. (A) Elastographic analysis of the tibial ACL-to-bone insertion (TI) under applied uniaxial tension. Displacement map calculated from ultrasound radiofrequency data (increase in magnitude: *blue* to *red*, bar = 5 mm). A region-dependent decrease in displacement is related to increase in tissue stiffness from the ligament to fibrocartilage interface and then to bone. (B) Energy dispersive X-ray analysis (EDAX) across the ACL-to-bone insertion revealed region-dependent changes in mineral content from the non-mineralized (NFC) to the mineralized fibrocartilage region (MFC) and to bone. Calcium (Ca, *blue*) and phosphorous (P, *red*) peaks are detected only within the MFC and bone regions; whereas the sulfur (S, *green*) peak intensity diminished from the NFC to the MFC region (200×, scale = 50 μm). (C) Correlation of Young's modulus and phosphorous peak intensity for the NFC and MFC regions of the ACL-to-bone insertion site. An increase in Young's modulus strongly correlates (R = 0.868) with higher phosphorous peak intensity, suggesting a structure–function relationship between insertion site mechanical properties and mineral distribution.

compressive strains were detected at the insertion while the knee was loaded in tension.

Direct measurement of interface mechanical properties has been difficult due to the complexity and the relative small scale of the interface, in general ranging from 100 μm to 1 mm in length.[1,3,43,73] Thus existing knowledge of insertion material properties has been largely derived from theoretic models.[41,69] Recently, Moffat and colleagues[6] performed the first experimental determination of the compressive mechanical properties of the ACL-to-bone interface. Specifically, the incremental displacement field of the fibrocartilage tissue under the applied uniaxial strain was evaluated by coupling micro-compression with optimized digital image correlation (DIC) analysis of the pre- and post-loading images.[74] Similar to the elastography findings,[72] deformation decreased gradually from the fibrocartilage interface to bone. Moreover, these region-dependent changes were accompanied by a gradual increase in compressive modulus. The interface also exhibited a region-dependent decrease in strain, with a significantly higher elastic modulus found in the mineralized fibrocartilage when compared with the non-mineralized region.[6] In the neonatal bovine model, the compressive modulus of the non-mineralized fibrocartilage region is 0.32 ± 0.14 MPa,[6] representing less than 50% of the mineralized fibrocartilage modulus (0.68 ± 0.39 MPa).[6] Both of these values are lower than that of trabecular bone, which is reported to be 173 ± 97 MPa in the same animal model.[75] These interface region-specific mechanical properties enable a gradual transition rather than an abrupt increase in tissue strain across the insertion and provide valuable cues for interface scaffold design.

Given the structure–function dependence inherent in the biological system, the regional changes in mechanical properties reported by Moffat and colleagues[6] are likely correlated to differences in matrix organization and composition across the interface. Partition of the fibrocartilage interface into non-mineralized and mineralized regions is anticipated to have a functional significance, because increases in matrix mineral content have been associated with higher mechanical properties in connective tissues.[76–78] Evaluation of the insertion site using Fourier Transform Infrared Imaging (FTIR-I, see **Fig. 1**B)[79] and X-ray analysis[6] revealed an increase in calcium and phosphorous content progressing from ligament, interface, and then to bone (see **Fig. 2**B). An abrupt transition, instead of a gradient of mineral distribution, was detected when transiting from the non-mineralized to the mineralized interface regions. Similar to other connective tissues,[35] this increase in elastic modulus progressing from the non-mineralized to the mineralized fibrocartilage interface region was shown to be positively correlated[6] with the presence of calcium phosphate (see **Fig. 2**C).

Elucidation of the structure–function relationship inherent at the ligament-to-bone insertion has yielded invaluable clues for the design of biomimetic scaffolds for regenerating this complex multi-tissue interface. The intricate multi-tissue organization and controlled matrix heterogeneity observed at the ACL-to-bone junction suggest that interface scaffold design must consider the need to regenerate more than 1 type of tissue as well as exercising spatial control over the respective cell populations indigenous to the ACL-to-bone interface regions. Additionally, a gradual increase in mechanical properties across the scaffold phases is needed to prevent the formation of stress concentrations. This may be achieved by regulating the distribution and concentration of calcium phosphate on the scaffold phases.

ROLE OF CELLULAR INTERACTIONS IN THE MECHANISM OF INTERFACE REGENERATION

As described above, the native ACL-to-bone insertion consists of a linear progression of 3 distinct matrix regions: ligament, fibrocartilage, and bone, with each region exhibiting a characteristic cellular phenotype and matrix composition. It is likely that communication among the 3 resident cell populations, namely fibroblasts, fibrochondrocytes and osteoblasts, is important for interface homeostasis and regeneration. The insertion fibrochondrocyte phenotype is not well defined because fibrocartilaginous tissues differ in composition and structure depending on the anatomic site.[23,80] Sun and colleagues[81] compared the response of fibrochondrocytes isolated directly from the ACL-to-bone insertion to those of inner- and outer-ring meniscal fibrochondrocytes as well as ligament fibroblasts and articular chondrocytes. It was found that the greatest increase in proteoglycan synthesis was detected in insertion fibrochondrocytes and articular chondrocytes. In addition, the fibrochondrocytes produced a matrix containing both type I and type II collagen. Cell alkaline phosphatase (ALP) activity peaked at 1 week for the insertion fibrochondrocytes and was significantly higher than that of articular chondrocytes or meniscal fibrochondrocytes. Aside from its mineralization potential, these findings suggest that the ACL insertion fibrochondrocytes appear to be similar to articular chondrocytes, while differing significantly from the meniscal fibrochondrocytes and ligament fibroblasts.

Currently, the mechanism of interface regeneration is not known. A fundamental question in interface tissue engineering is how distinct boundaries between different types of connective tissues are reestablished post-injury. When Fujioka and colleagues[82] sutured the Achilles tendon to its original attachment site, cellular organization resembling that of the native insertion and the deposition of collagen type X were observed in vivo. It is also well established that although tendon-to-bone healing following ACL reconstruction does not lead to the re-establishment of the native insertion, a layer of fibrocartilage-like tissue is formed within the bone tunnel.[11,57,83] These observations collectively suggest that when trauma or injury to the interface results in non-physiologic exposure of normally segregated tissue types (eg, bone, ligament, or tendon), interactions between the resident cell populations in these tissues (osteoblast-fibroblast) are likely critical for initiating and directing the repair response that leads to the re-establishment of a fibrocartilage interface between soft tissue and bone. In vivo cell-tracking studies have also revealed that the tendon graft is usually invaded by host cells within 1 week of implantation,[84] indicating that cell types other than the osteoblasts and fibroblasts populating the graft-bone junction may be involved in fibrocartilage regeneration. Based on these observations, Lu and Jiang[7] proposed a working hypothesis for interface regeneration, suggesting that osteoblast–fibroblast interactions mediate interface regeneration through heterotypic cellular interactions, which can lead to phenotypic changes or trans-differentiation of osteoblasts and/or fibroblasts. In addition, these interactions can promote the differentiation of stem cells or progenitor cells into fibrochondrocytes and promote the regeneration of the fibrocartilage interface.

Several in vitro studies evaluating the role of heterotypic cellular interactions on interface regeneration have been reported.[85,86] Co-culture and tri-culture models of interface-relevant cell populations were used to determine the effects of cellular communication on the development of fibrocartilage-specific markers in vitro. Wang and colleagues[85] examined the interaction between osteoblasts and ligament fibroblasts, whereby a 2-D co-culture model, permitting both cell physical contact and soluble factor interactions, was designed to emulate the in vivo condition in which the tendon graft is in direct contact with bone tissue following ACL reconstruction (**Fig. 3**A, inset). Osteoblasts and fibroblasts were first separated by a hydrogel divider, and on reaching confluence, the divider was removed, allowing the osteoblasts and fibroblasts to migrate and interact directly within the interface region (see **Fig. 3**A). It was reported that these controlled interactions decreased cell proliferation (see **Fig. 3**B), altered the

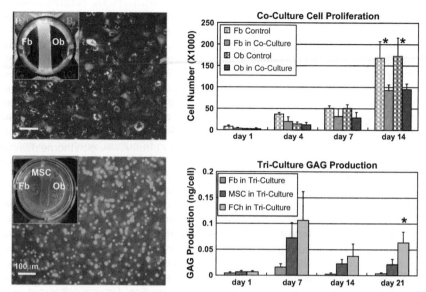

Fig. 3. Co-culture and Tri-Culture Models for Evaluating the Interaction between Interface-Relevant Cell Populations. In vitro co-culture model of fibroblasts (Fb) and osteoblasts (Ob) (inset) and the cellular interactions between Fb (CM-DiI) and Ob (CFDA-SE) in co-culture (bar = 100 μm). Co-culture modulated the proliferation of fibroblasts and osteoblasts (*P < .05). In vitro tri-culture model (inset) to evaluate the effects of osteoblast–fibroblast interactions on the fibrochondrogenic differentiation of bone marrow-derived mesenchymal stem cells (MSC) and ligament fibroblasts (Fb). Insertion fibrochondrocytes (FCh) served as the positive control. (Live-dead stain, MSC in hydrogel, d 40, bar = 100 μm). Co-culture modulated glycosaminoglycan (GAG) production by interface-relevant cells (Fb, MSC, FCh) (*P < 0.05).

ALP activity profile, and promoted the expression of matrix proteins characteristic of the fibrocartilage interface, such as types I and II collagen, and cartilage oligomeric matrix protein (COMP). Subsequent conditioned media studies have revealed that both autocrine and paracrine factors were responsible for the changes in phenotype observed during osteoblast-fibroblast co-culture.[87] Although it is unknown which or if any of the two 2 populations are directly responsible for interface regeneration, these observations suggest that osteoblast–fibroblast interactions are key modulators of cell phenotype at the graft-to-bone junction. These cellular interactions will certainly have a downstream effect, either in terms of inducing cell trans-differentiation into fibrochondrocytes or in the recruitment and differentiation of progenitor or stem cells for fibrocartilage formation.

Although osteoblast–fibroblast interactions resulted in phenotypic changes and the expression of interface-relevant markers in co-culture, a fibrocartilage-like interface was not formed in vitro. Recently, when Lim and colleagues[88] coated tendon grafts with mesenchymal stem cells embedded in a fibrin gel, the formation of a zone of cartilaginous tissue between graft and bone was observed, suggesting a potential role for stem cells in fibrocartilage formation. Thus, other cell types such as fibrochondrocyte precursors or stem cells may be involved in interface regeneration, and it is likely that osteoblast–fibroblast interactions may direct the fibrochondrogenic differentiation of these cells. In addition, the insertion site is derived from the ligament during development,[38,39,89,90] and dermal fibroblasts as well as cells residing in tendon or ligament have been shown to exhibit fibrochondrocyte- or chondrocyte-like phenotype under controlled conditions.[91–94] Building on the 2-D co-culture model, Wang and colleagues[95] designed a tri-culture system (see **Fig. 3**C, inset) of fibroblasts, osteoblasts, and interface-relevant cell populations, such as fibroblasts and bone marrow-derived mesenchymal stem cells (MSC). The response of MSC or fibroblasts in tri-culture was compared with those of ACL-to-bone insertion fibrochondrocytes or articular chondrocytes maintained under similar conditions. In tri-culture, fibroblasts and osteoblasts were each seeded on cover slips on the opposite sides of the well, with either fibroblasts or MSC pre-loaded into the hydrogel insert. In addition to being able to assess the response of individual cell types in tri-culture, another advantage of this model system is that physiologically relevant 3-D instead of monolayer culture can be maintained at the interface region (see **Fig. 3**C).

Under the influence of osteoblast–fibroblast interactions, it was found that cell number for the MSC, fibrochondrocyte, and articular chondrocyte groups remained relatively constant, whereas ligament fibroblasts proliferated readily in tri-culture. Unlike fibroblasts, MSC in tri-culture exhibited a level of ALP activity similar to that of insertion fibrochondrocytes, with both groups peaking by day 7 and decreasing thereafter. In addition, while minimal proteoglycan deposition was seen in the fibroblast group, MSC measured significantly higher proteoglycan synthesis in tri-culture, although the level of response was lower than that of insertion fibrochondrocytes (see **Fig. 3**D). Moreover, under stimulation by osteoblast–fibroblast interactions, both insertion fibrochondrocytes and MSC produced a type II collagen-containing matrix, whereas no such matrix was observed for fibroblasts following tri-culture.

The multi-scale co-culture and tri-culture systems described here are simple and elegant models that can be used to systematically investigate the mechanisms governing interface regeneration. Findings from the reported in vitro studies of heterotypic cellular interactions provide preliminary validation of the hypothesis that osteoblast–fibroblast interactions play a regulatory role in the induction of interface-specific markers in progenitor or stem cells and demonstrate the effects of heterotypic cellular interactions in regulating the maintenance of soft tissue-to-bone junctions. Although the mechanisms of interaction and the nature of the regulatory cytokines secreted remain elusive, cell communication is likely to be significant for interface regeneration and homeostasis. Therefore, the optimal interface scaffold must promote interactions between the relevant cell populations residing in each interface region.

STRATIFIED SCAFFOLD FOR LIGAMENT–BONE INTERFACE TISSUE ENGINEERING

Investigations of the interface structure–function relationships as well as the role of cellular interactions in interface regeneration have provided invaluable insight into biomimetic scaffold design for orthopedic interface tissue engineering. The multi-tissue transition (ligament, fibrocartilage, bone) represents a significant challenge because several distinct yet contiguous tissue regions constitute the complex insertion site. A stratified scaffold design will, therefore, be essential for recapturing the aforementioned complexity of the native ligament-to-bone interface. The ideal scaffold for interface tissue engineering, in addition to supporting the growth and differentiation of relevant cell populations, must also direct heterotypic and homotypic cellular interactions while promoting the formation and maintenance of controlled matrix heterogeneity. Consequently, the scaffold should exhibit a gradient of structural and mechanical properties mimicking those of the native insertion site. Compared with a homogenous structure, a scaffold with pre-designed, tissue-specific matrix inhomogeneity can better sustain and transmit the distribution of complex loads inherent at the ACL-to-bone interface. It is emphasized that while the scaffold is stratified or consisted of different phases, a key criterion is that these phases must be interconnected and pre-integrated with one an other, thereby supporting the formation of distinct yet continuous multi-tissue regions. The interface scaffold must also possess mechanical properties comparable to those of the ligament-to-bone interface. In addition, the scaffold phases should be biodegradable so that it is gradually replaced by living tissue, although its degradation must be controlled to sustain physiologic loading and promote neo-interface function. Finally, for in vivo graft integration, the interface scaffold must be easily adaptable with current ACL reconstruction grafts or pre-incorporated into the design of ligament replacement grafts.

Traditional efforts in synthetic or tissue engineered alternatives for ACL reconstruction have focused on regenerating the ligament proper.[30,32,96] Recently, a more complex design of a synthetic ACL graft, consisting of a ligament proper and 2 bony regions,[33,34] was fabricated by 3-D braiding of polylactide-co-glycolide (PLGA) fibers, with the extended goal of promoting ACL graft integration within the bone tunnels. In vitro[34] and in vivo[97] evaluations demonstrated biocompatibility, healing, and long-term mechanical strength in a rabbit model. Although the strength of the ligament region is necessary for the success of the ACL graft, establishment of a stable graft-to-bone interface will also be critical for the long-term functionality of the tissue engineered graft. Recently, Spalazzi and colleagues[98,99] reported on the design and evaluation of a tri-phasic scaffold (see **Fig. 1**C) for the regeneration of the ACL-to-bone interface. Modeled after the multi-tissue native insertion site, the scaffold consists of 3 distinct yet continuous phases, each pre-engineered for a particular interface cell population and tissue region: Phase A is designed with a PLGA (10:90) mesh for fibroblast culture and soft tissue formation, Phase B consists of PLGA (85:15) microspheres and is the interface region intended for fibrochondrocyte culture, and Phase C is composed of sintered PLGA (85:15) and 45S5 bioactive glass composite microspheres[18] for osteoblast culture and bone formation. It is noted that the innovative stratified scaffold design and fabrication method resulted in essence in a "single" scaffold system with 3 distinct yet continuous phases, intended to support the formation of the multi-tissue regions observed across the ACL-bone junction.

Interactions between interface relevant cell populations (eg, fibroblasts, chondrocytes, and osteoblasts) on the tri-phasic scaffold have been evaluated both in vitro and in vivo.[98–100] For co-culture, human ligament fibroblasts and osteoblasts were seeded on Phase A and Phase C, respectively,[98] whereas Phase B was left unseeded. The migration of both cell types into Phase B was monitored over time. It was observed that fibroblasts and osteoblasts were localized primarily at opposite ends of the scaffolds post-seeding, with few cells found in Phase B. After 4 weeks, each cell type proliferated within their respective phases as well as migrated into Phase B. The stratified scaffold design promoted phase-specific cell distribution, with osteoblasts and fibroblasts localized in their respective regions, whereas their interaction was restricted to Phase B, the interface region (see **Fig. 1**D). Spatial control over cell distribution also resulted in the elaboration of a cell type-specific matrix on each phase of the scaffold, with a mineralized matrix detected only on Phase C and an extensive type I collagen matrix found on both Phases A and B. When the tri-phasic scaffold co-cultured with osteoblasts and fibroblasts was evaluated in a subcutaneous athymic rat model,[99,100] abundant tissue formation was observed on Phases A and C. Cells migrated into Phase B, and increased matrix production was found in this interface region. Moreover, tissue continuity was maintained across all 3 scaffold phases. Interestingly, extracellular matrix production compensated for the decrease in mechanical properties accompanying scaffold degradation, and phase-specific controlled matrix heterogeneity was maintained in vivo.

Similar to the findings of the 2-D co-culture model, although both anatomic ligament- and bone-like matrices were formed on the tri-phasic scaffold in vitro and in vivo, no fibrocartilage-like tissue was observed within the interface phase through osteoblast-fibroblast co-culture. Spalazzi and colleagues[99] extended their in vivo evaluation to tri-culture of fibroblasts, chondrocytes, and osteoblasts on the stratified scaffold. Articular chondrocytes encapsulated in a hydrogel matrix were injected into Phase B of the scaffold, whereas fibroblasts and osteoblasts were seeded onto Phases A and C, respectively. At 2 months post-implantation, an extensive collagen-rich matrix was prevalent in all 3 phases of the tri-cultured scaffolds (see **Fig. 1E**), and the mineralized matrix was again confined to Phase C. The fibrocartilage region formed in tri-culture exhibited characteristic markers, such as types I and II collagen as well as proteoglycan production. Interestingly, both cell shape and matrix morphology of the neo-fibrocartilage resembled that of the neonatal fibrocartilage tissue observed at the ACL-bone insertion.[3] Moreover, the neo-fibrocartilage formed was continuous with the ligament-like tissue observed in Phase A as well as the bone-like tissue found in Phase C.[100]

These promising results demonstrate that biomimetic stratified scaffold design coupled with spatial control over the distribution of interface-relevant cell populations leads to the formation of cell type- and phase-specific matrix heterogeneity in vitro and in vivo, with a fibrocartilage-like interface formed in tri-culture. These observations not only demonstrate the feasibility of the stratified scaffold for promoting biological fixation but also highlight the potential for continuous multi-tissue regeneration on a single scaffold system. It is envisioned that the tri-phasic scaffold can be used to guide the re-establishment of an anatomic fibrocartilage interfacial region directly on soft tissue grafts. Specifically, the scaffold can be used as a graft collar or a circumferential interference screw during ACL reconstruction surgery. As a graft collar, it can be fabricated as a hollow cylinder through which the ACL graft is inserted, seeded with interface-relevant cells on each phase, and secured to the ends of the graft. It is anticipated that the phase-specific matrix heterogeneity and optimized cellular interactions, combined with application of both mechanical and chemical stimuli, would be able to induce the formation of a fibrocartilage interface directly onto the soft tissue graft. For use as an interference screw, the tri-phasic scaffold can be fabricated as matching halves of a hollow cylinder, with each half containing the 3 scaffold phases. The 2 matching halves encase the soft tissue graft on all sides. The relative position of each phase of the tri-phasic scaffold would be in the anatomic position, that is, with Phase A (soft tissue) exposed to the joint cavity, Phase B (fibrocartilage interface) flush with articular cartilage, and Phase C (bone) encased within the bone tunnel. The feasibility of such a system for interface regeneration was recently demonstrated in a study by Spalazzi and colleagues,[101] where a mechanoactive scaffold system was formed based on a composite of poly-α-hydroxyester nanofibers and sintered microspheres. It was observed that scaffold-induced compression of tendon grafts resulted in significant matrix remodeling and the expression of fibrocartilage interface-related markers such as type II collagen, aggrecan, and transforming growth factor-$\beta 3$ (TGF-$\beta 3$). These results demonstrate that the stratified scaffold can be used to induce the formation of an anatomic fibrocartilage enthesis directly on ACL reconstruction grafts.

It is emphasized here that fixation of the aforementioned graft collar or interference screw is achieved by inserting the collar-graft complex into the bone tunnel, with Phases A and B remaining within the joint cavity. The ACL graft can also be augmented with mechanical fixation until an anatomic interface has been regenerated on the graft. Controlled cellular interactions coupled with mechanical loading may promote the formation of a fibrocartilage region directly on the ACL reconstruction graft. In parallel, graft osteointegration within the bone tunnel may be promoted by Phase C and the delivery of growth factors (eg, bone morphogenetic proteins)[58,102–104] to stimulate tendon mineralization within the bone tunnel. The optimal scenario is to have a completely mineralized tendon within the bone tunnel, accompanied by the formation of an anatomic fibrocartilage insertion directly on the ACL reconstruction graft. In addition, for functional ligament tissue engineering, the tri-phasic scaffold may be coupled with synthetic ACL grafts either as a graft collar or pre-incorporated into degradable polymer-based ACL prostheses.[34] It is anticipated that by focusing on engineering soft tissue-to-bone integration ex vivo, the complexity of intra-articular graft reconstruction would be reduced to bone-to-bone integration in vivo, which may be relatively less challenging when compared with soft tissue-to-bone integration.

STRATIFIED SCAFFOLD FOR TENDON–BONE INTERFACE TISSUE ENGINEERING

Because soft tissue-to-bone interfaces are ubiquitous in the musculoskeletal system, the biomimetic scaffold design and multi-lineage cell culture methods described above are applicable to the regeneration of other soft tissue-to-bone insertions, such as that of the rotator cuff tendons and bone. Similar to the ACL insertion site, a zonal distribution of extracellular matrix components and cell types is found at the supraspinatus tendon-to-bone interface.[2,41,43,105,106] Additionally, the repair of the supraspinatus tendon is characterized by disorganized scar tissue and the lack of fibrocartilage regeneration at the insertion site.[107,108] The debilitating effect of rotator cuff tears coupled with the high incidence of failure associated with existing repair techniques[109–112] underscores the clinical need for functional solutions for supraspinatus tendon-to-bone repair.

Several groups have evaluated the feasibility of integrating tendon grafts with bone or biomaterials through the formation of anatomic insertion sites.[82,113] Fujioka and colleagues[82] reported that cellular reorganization occurred at the site of surgical reattachment of the Achilles tendon, along with the formation of non-mineralized and mineralized fibrocartilage-like regions. Additionally, Inoue and colleagues[82,113] used a bone marrow-infused bone graft to promote supraspinatus tendon integration with a metallic implant. Promising results from these early studies demonstrate that the tendon-bone interface may be regenerated and emphasize the need for functional grafting solutions that can promote biological fixation. The ideal scaffold for supraspinatus tendon repair must be able to meet the physiologic demand of the native tendon by matching its mechanical properties as well as promoting host cell-mediated healing by mimicking the ultrastructural organization of the native tendon. In addition, the scaffold should be biodegradable in order to be gradually replaced by new tissue while maintaining physiologically relevant mechanical properties. Finally, the scaffold must be able to integrate with the host tendon and surrounding bone tissue by promoting the regeneration of the native tendon-to-bone enthesis.

Guided by these design criteria, the potential of a degradable PLGA nanofiber-based scaffold system (**Fig. 4**) for rotator cuff repair was recently evaluated in vitro.[28] Nanofibers are advantageous for orthopedic tissue engineering due to their superior biomimetic potential and physiologic relevance. To date, nanofibers have been investigated for bone,[114,115] meniscus,[116] intervertebral disk,[117] cartilage,[118] and ligament[119,120] tissue engineering. A distinct advantage of nanofiber scaffolds is that they can be tailored to resemble the native tendon extracellular matrix, exhibiting high aspect ratio, surface area, permeability, and porosity.[121–125] Moreover, nanofiber organization and alignment can be modulated during fabrication,[125,126] which allows

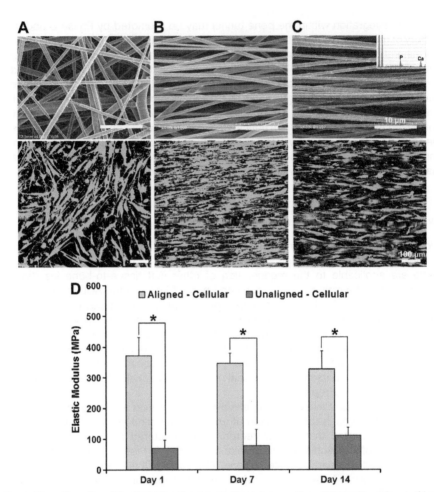

Fig. 4. Nanofiber-Based Scaffold for Tendon-to-Bone Integration. (*A*) Unaligned nanofibers based on PLGA supported the attachment and growth of human rotator cuff tendon fibroblasts (*Top*, as-fabricated scaffold, bar = 10 μm; *Bottom*, Live-dead stain, d 14, 20×, bar = 100 μm). (*B*) Aligned PLGA nanofibers guided the alignment of human rotator cuff tendon fibroblasts (*Top*, as-fabricated scaffold, bar = 10 μm; *Bottom*, Live-dead stain, d 14, 20×, bar = 100 μm). (*C*) Nanofiber composite of PLGA and hydroxyapatite particles also supported tendon fibroblast growth and alignment (*Top*, as-fabricated scaffold with HA particles (inset), bar = 10 μm; *Bottom*, Live-dead stain, d 14, 20×, bar = 100 μm). (*D*) Mechanical properties of the aligned and unaligned nanofiber scaffolds seeded with supraspinatus tendon fibroblasts as a function of in vitro culture time (*$P < 0.05$).

the structural and material properties of the scaffold to be readily tailored to meet the functional demands of the rotator cuff tendons.

Recently, the effects of nanofiber organization on cellular attachment and alignment as well as gene expression and matrix deposition were evaluated.[28] It was reported that nanofiber organization (aligned versus unaligned) is the primary factor guiding tendon fibroblast morphology (see **Fig. 4**), alignment, and integrin expression. Moreover, both types I and III collagen, the primary collagen types found in the native supraspinatus tendon, were synthesized on the nanofiber scaffolds and, interestingly, their deposition was also controlled by the underlying fiber organization. Scaffold mechanical properties are directly related to fiber alignment and although they decreased as the polymer degraded, both the elastic modulus (see **Fig. 4**) and ultimate tensile strength remain within range of those reported for the native supraspinatus tendon.[127]

Building on the aligned nanofiber system, Moffat and colleagues[128] later designed a composite nanofiber system of PLGA and hydroxyapatite (HA) nanoparticles, with the extended goal of regenerating both the non-mineralized and mineralized fibrocartilage regions of the supraspinatus tendon-to-bone insertion site. The response of interface-relevant cell populations, including rotator cuff fibroblasts and osteoblasts, has been examined on the polymer-ceramic composite nanofibers with promising results (see **Fig. 4C**). These observations demonstrate the potential of the biodegradable nanofiber-based scaffold system for tendon tissue engineering and underscore the need for the development of stratified scaffolds for integrative rotator cuff repair and augmentation.

SUMMARY AND CHALLENGES IN INTERFACE TISSUE ENGINEERING

Interface tissue engineering focuses on the regeneration of the anatomic interface between distinct tissue types and has the potential to provide integrative graft solutions that will expedite the translation of tissue engineered technologies to the clinical setting. Building on the solid foundation of tissue engineering methods already validated in past studies, interface tissue engineering aims to develop innovative technologies for the formation of complex tissue systems, with the extended goal of achieving the *biological* fixation of tissue engineered grafts with each other and with the host environment. Current efforts in this emerging area have centered on the formation of a functional interface between distinct tissue types, guided by the working hypothesis that tissue interfaces may be regenerated from the controlled interaction of relevant cell types on a biomimetic stratified scaffold with a pre-designed gradient of structural and functional properties.

The broader question to be addressed in orthopedic interface tissue engineering is how distinct boundaries between different types of connective tissues are formed, re-established post-injury, and maintained in the body. The success of any interface tissue engineering effort will require a thorough understanding of the structure–function relationship existing at the native insertion site and the elucidation of the mechanisms governing interface regeneration and homeostasis. Although most research has focused on interface formation, the engineering of multiple tissue types must also address the problem of maintaining the stability of pre-formed tissue regions. It is likely that heterotypic cellular interactions will also play a critical role in interface homeostasis.[129] Moreover, the effects of biological, physical, and chemical stimulation on interface regeneration are not known and remain to be explored.

In summary, the re-establishment of an anatomic, functional, and stable interface on biologic or synthetic soft tissue grafts through interface tissue engineering represents a promising strategy for achieving biological graft fixation for ligament or tendon reconstruction and augmenting the clinical translation potential of tissue engineered orthopedic grafts. The multi-phasic scaffold design principles and coculturing methodologies optimized through these efforts can lead to the development of a new generation of integrative fixation devices for orthopedic repairs. Moreover, by bridging distinct types of tissue, interface tissue engineering will be instrumental for the ex vivo development and in vivo translation of integrated musculoskeletal tissue systems with biomimetic complexity and functionality.

ACKNOWLEDGMENTS

The authors gratefully acknowledge the contribution of all students, fellows, and collaborators who have worked on the orthopedic interface tissue engineering research described in this review. We also thank the National Institutes of Health (NIH/NIAMS AR052402, HHL; AR056459, HHL; and AR055280-A2, HHL/SAR), the Wallace H. Coulter Foundation (HHL/SAR), and the National Science Foundation GK-12 Graduate Fellowship (GK-12 0,338,329, KLM) for funding support.

REFERENCES

1. Cooper RR, Misol S. Tendon and ligament insertion. A light and electron micro-scopic study. J Bone Joint Surg Am 1970;52:1–20.
2. Benjamin M, Evano EJ, Copp L. The histology of tendon attachments to bone in man. J Anat 1986;149:89–100.
3. Wang IE, Mitroo S, Chen FH, et al. Age-dependent changes in matrix composi-tion and organization at the ligament-to-bone insertion. J Orthop Res 2006;24: 1745–55.
4. Woo SL, Maynard J, Butler DL, et al. Ligament, tendon, and joint capsule inser-tions to bone. In: Woo SL, Bulkwater JA, editors. Injury and repair of the muscu-losketal soft tissues. Savannah (GA): American Academy of Orthopaedic Surgeons; 1988. p. 133–66.
5. Woo SL, Gomez MA, Seguchi Y, et al. Measurement of mechanical properties of ligament substance from a bone-ligament-bone preparation. J Orthop Res 1983; 1:22–9.
6. Moffat KL, Sun WH, Pena PE, et al. Characterization of the structure-function re-lationship at the ligament-to-bone interface. Proc Natl Acad Sci USA 2008;105: 7947–52.
7. Lu HH, Jiang J. Interface tissue engineering and the formulation of multiple-tissue systems. Adv Biochem Eng Biotechnol 2006;102:91–111.
8. Friedman MJ, Sherman OH, Fox JM, et al. Autogeneic anterior cruciate ligament (ACL) anterior reconstruction of the knee. A review. Clin Orthop 1985;196:9–14.
9. Kurosaka M, Yoshiya S, Andrish JT. A biomechanical comparison of different sur-gical techniques of graft fixation in anterior cruciate ligament reconstruction. Am J Sports Med 1987;15:225–9.
10. Robertson DB, Daniel DM, Biden E. Soft tissue fixation to bone. Am J Sports Med 1986;14:398–403.
11. Rodeo SA, Arnoczky SP, Torzilli PA, et al. Tendon-healing in a bone tunnel. A bio-mechanical and histological study in the dog. J Bone Joint Surg Am 1993;75: 1795–803.
12. Skalak R. Tissue engineering. Proceedings of the UCLA Symposium on Molec-ular and Cellular Biology. Lake Tahoe, California, February 26–29, 1988.
13. Langer R, Vacanti JP. Tissue engineering. Science 1993;260:920–6.
14. Mikos AG, Sarakinos G, Leite SM, et al. Laminated three-dimensional biode-gradable foams for use in tissue engineering. Biomaterials 1993;14:323–30.
15. Yaszemski MJ, Payne RG, Hayes WC, et al. Evolution of bone transplantation: molecular, cellular and tissue strategies to engineer human bone. Biomaterials 1996;17:175–85.
16. Laurencin CT, Ambrosio AA, Borden M, et al. Tissue engineering: orthopedic applications. In: Yarmush ML, Diller KR, Toner M, editors. Annual review of biomedical engineering. Palo Alto (CA): Annual Reviews; 1999. p. 19–46.

17. Agrawal CM, Ray RB. Biodegradable polymeric scaffolds for musculoskeletal tissue engineering. J Biomed Mater Res 2001;55:141–50.
18. Lu HH, El Amin SF, Scott KD, et al. Three-dimensional, bioactive, biodegradable, polymer-bioactive glass composite scaffolds with improved mechanical properties support collagen synthesis and mineralization of human osteoblast-like cells in vitro. J Biomed Mater Res 2003;64A:465–74.
19. Freed LE, Marquis JC, Nohria A, et al. Neocartilage formation in vitro and in vivo using cells cultured on synthetic biodegradable polymers. J Biomed Mater Res 1993;27:11–23.
20. Vunjak-Novakovic G, Freed LE, Biron RJ, et al. Effects of mixing on the composition and morphology of tissue- engineered cartilage. AIChE J 1996; 42:850–60.
21. Mauck RL, Soltz MA, Wang CC, et al. Functional tissue engineering of articular cartilage through dynamic loading of chondrocyte-seeded agarose gels. J Biomech Eng 2000;122:252–60.
22. Lu L, Zhu X, Valenzuela RG, et al. Biodegradable polymer scaffolds for cartilage tissue engineering. Clin Orthop 2001;391:S251–70.
23. Almarza AJ, Athanasiou KA. Design characteristics for the tissue engineering of cartilaginous tissues. Ann Biomed Eng 2004;32:2–17.
24. Garvin J, Qi J, Maloney M, et al. Novel system for engineering bioartificial tendons and application of mechanical load. Tissue Eng 2003;9:967–79.
25. Zhang AY, Chang J. Tissue engineering of flexor tendons. Clin Plast Surg 2003; 30:565–72.
26. Goh JC, Ouyang HW, Teoh SH, et al. Tissue-engineering approach to the repair and regeneration of tendons and ligaments. Tissue Eng 2003;9:S31–44.
27. Juncosa N, West JR, Galloway MT, et al. In vivo forces used to develop design parameters for tissue engineered implants for rabbit patellar tendon repair. J Biomech 2003;36:483–8.
28. Moffat KL, Spalazzi JP, Doty SB, et al Novel nanofiber-based scaffold for rotator cuff repair and augmentation. Tissue Eng 2008 [epub ahead of print].
29. Jackson DW, Heinrich JT, Simon TM. Biologic and synthetic implants to replace the anterior cruciate ligament. Arthroscopy 1994;10:442–52.
30. Dunn MG, Liesch JB, Tiku ML, et al. Development of fibroblast-seeded ligament analogs for ACL reconstruction. J Biomed Mater Res 1995;29:1363–71.
31. Woo SL, Hildebrand K, Watanabe N, et al. Tissue engineering of ligament and tendon healing. Clin Orthop Relat Res 1999;367:S312–23.
32. Altman GH, Horan RL, Lu HH, et al. Silk matrix for tissue engineered anterior cruciate ligaments. Biomaterials 2002;23:4131–41.
33. Cooper JA, Lu HH, Ko FK, et al. Fiber-based tissue-engineered scaffold for ligament replacement: design considerations and in vitro evaluation. Biomaterials 2005;26:1523–32.
34. Lu HH, Cooper JA, Manuel S, et al. Anterior cruciate ligament regeneration using braided biodegradable scaffolds: in vitro optimization studies. Biomaterials 2005;26:4805–16.
35. Benjamin M, Evans EJ, Rao RD, et al. Quantitative differences in the histology of the attachment zones of the meniscal horns in the knee joint of man. J Anat 1991;177:127–34.
36. Niyibizi C, Visconti CS, Kavalkovich K, et al. Collagens in an adult bovine medial collateral ligament: immunofluorescence localization by confocal microscopy reveals that type XIV collagen predominates at the ligament-bone junction. Matrix Biol 1995;14:743–51.

37. Sagarriga VC, Kavalkovich K, Wu J, et al. Biochemical analysis of collagens at the ligament-bone interface reveals presence of cartilage-specific collagens. Arch Biochem Biophys 1996;328:135–42.
38. Wei X, Messner K. The postnatal development of the insertions of the medial collateral ligament in the rat knee. Anat Embryol (Berl) 1996;193:53–9.
39. Messner K. Postnatal development of the cruciate ligament insertions in the rat knee. Morphological evaluation and immunohistochemical study of collagens types I and II. Acta Anatomica 1997;160:261–8.
40. Petersen W, Tillmann B. Structure and vascularization of the cruciate ligaments of the human knee joint. Anat Embryol (Berl) 1999;200:325–34.
41. Thomopoulos S, Williams GR, Gimbel JA, et al. Variations of biomechanical, structural, and compositional properties along the tendon to bone insertion site. J Orthop Res 2003;21:413–9.
42. Niyibizi C, Sagarriga VC, Gibson G, et al. Identification and immunolocalization of type X collagen at the ligament-bone interface. Biochem Biophys Res Commun 1996;222:584–9.
43. Woo SL, Buckwalter JA. Injury and repair of the musculoskeletal soft tissues. J Orthop Res 1988;6:907–31.
44. Johnson RJ. The anterior cruciate: a dilemma in sports medicine. Int J Sports Med 1982;3:71–9.
45. American Academy of Orthopaedic Surgeons. How old is too old to repair the ACL? [press release]; 2008.
46. Gotlin RS, Huie G. Anterior cruciate ligament injuries. Operative and rehabilitative options. Phys Med Rehabil Clin N Am 2000;11:895–928.
47. Fleming BC, Abate JA, Peura GD, et al. The relationship between graft tensioning and the anterior-posterior laxity in the anterior cruciate ligament reconstructed goat knee. J Orthop Res 2001;19:841–4.
48. Fleming B, Beynnon B, Howe J, et al. Effect of tension and placement of a prosthetic anterior cruciate ligament on the anteroposterior laxity of the knee. J Orthop Res 1992;10:177–86.
49. Beynnon B, Yu J, Huston D, et al. A sagittal plane model of the knee and cruciate ligaments with application of a sensitivity analysis. J Biomech Eng 1996;118:227–39.
50. Beynnon BD, Johnson JR, Fleming BC, et al. The effect of functional knee bracing on the anterior cruciate ligament in the weightbearing and nonweightbearing knee. Am J Sports Med 1997;25:353–9.
51. Gregor RJ, Abelew TA. Tendon force measurements and movement control: a review. Med Sci Sports Exerc 1994;26:1359–72.
52. Loh JC, Fukuda Y, Tsuda E, et al. Knee stability and graft function following anterior cruciate ligament reconstruction: comparison between 11 o'clock and 10 o'clock femoral tunnel placement. Arthroscopy 2003;19:297–304.
53. Markolf KL, Hame S, Hunter DM, et al. Effects of femoral tunnel placement on knee laxity and forces in an anterior cruciate ligament graft. J Orthop Res 2002;20:1016–24.
54. Brand J Jr, Weiler A, Caborn DN, et al. Graft fixation in cruciate ligament reconstruction. Am J Sports Med 2000;28:761–74.
55. Beynnon BD, Johnson RJ, Fleming BC, et al. Anterior cruciate ligament replacement: comparison of bone-patellar tendon-bone grafts with two-strand hamstring grafts. A prospective, randomized study. J Bone Joint Surg Am 2002;84:1503–13.
56. Barrett GR, Noojin FK, Hartzog CW, et al. Reconstruction of the anterior cruciate ligament in females: a comparison of hamstring versus patellar tendon autograft. Arthroscopy 2002;18:46–54.

57. Blickenstaff KR, Grana WA, Egle D. Analysis of a semitendinosus autograft in a rabbit model. Am J Sports Med 1997;25:554–9.
58. Rodeo SA, Suzuki K, Deng XH, et al. Use of recombinant human bone morphogenetic protein-2 to enhance tendon healing in a bone tunnel. Am J Sports Med 1999;27:476–88.
59. Berg EE. Autograft bone-patella tendon-bone plug comminution with loss of ligament fixation and stability. Arthroscopy 1996;12:232–5.
60. Matthews LS, Soffer SR. Pitfalls in the use of interference screws for anterior cruciate ligament reconstruction: brief report. Arthroscopy 1989;5:225–6.
61. Kurzweil PR, Frogameni AD, Jackson DW. Tibial interference screw removal following anterior cruciate ligament reconstruction. Arthroscopy 1995;11:289–91.
62. Burkart A, Imhoff AB, Roscher E. Foreign-body reaction to the bioabsorbable suretac device. Arthroscopy 2000;16:91–5.
63. Allum RL. BASK Instructional Lecture 1: graft selection in anterior cruciate ligament reconstruction. Knee 2001;8:69–72.
64. Shellock FG, Mink JH, Curtin S, et al. MR imaging and metallic implants for anterior cruciate ligament reconstruction: assessment of ferromagnetism and artifact. J Magn Reson Imaging 1992;2:225–8.
65. Weiler A, Peine R, Pashmineh-Azar A, et al. Tendon healing in a bone tunnel. Part I: biomechanical results after biodegradable interference fit fixation in a model of anterior cruciate ligament reconstruction in sheep. Arthroscopy 2002;18:113–23.
66. Beynnon BD, Meriam CM, Ryder SH, et al. The effect of screw insertion torque on tendons fixed with spiked washers. Am J Sports Med 1998;26:536–9.
67. Jackson DW, Grood ES, Arnoczky SP, et al. Cruciate reconstruction using freeze dried anterior cruciate ligament allograft and a ligament augmentation device (LAD). An experimental study in a goat model. Am J Sports Med 1987;15:528–38.
68. Yahia L. Ligaments and Ligamentoplasties. Heidelberg (Berlin): Springer Verlag; 1997.
69. Matyas JR, Anton MG, Shrive NG, et al. Stress governs tissue phenotype at the femoral insertion of the rabbit MCL. J Biomech 1995;28:147–57.
70. Benjamin M, Ralphs JR. Fibrocartilage in tendons and ligaments–an adaptation to compressive load. J Anat 1998;193(Pt 4):481–94.
71. Konofagou EE, Ophir J. Precision estimation and imaging of normal and shear components of the 3D strain tensor in elastography. Phys Med Biol 2000;45:1553–63.
72. Spalazzi JP, Gallina J, Fung-Kee-Fung SD, et al. Elastographic imaging of strain distribution in the anterior cruciate ligament and at the ligament-bone insertions. J Orthop Res 2006;24:2001–10.
73. Gao J, Messner K. Quantitative comparison of soft tissue-bone interface at chondral ligament insertions in the rabbit knee joint. J Anat 1996;188:367–73.
74. Wang CC, Hung CT, Mow VC. An analysis of the effects of depth-dependent aggregate modulus on articular cartilage stress-relaxation behavior in compression. J Biomech 2001;34:75–84.
75. Swartz DE, Wittenberg RH, Shea M, et al. Physical and mechanical properties of calf lumbosacral trabecular bone. J Biomech 1991;24:1059–68.
76. Currey JD. The effect of porosity and mineral content on the Young's modulus of elasticity of compact bone. J Biomech 1988;21:131–9.
77. Ferguson VL, Bushby AJ, Boyde A. Nanomechanical properties and mineral concentration in articular calcified cartilage and subchondral bone. J Anat 2003;203:191–202.

78. Radhakrishnan P, Lewis NT, Mao JJ. Zone-specific micromechanical properties of the extracellular matrices of growth plate cartilage. Ann Biomed Eng 2004;32: 284–91.

79. Spalazzi JP, Boskey AL, Lu HH. Region-dependent variations in matrix collagen and mineral distribution across the femoral and tibial anterior cruciate ligament-to-bone insertion sites [abstract 0891]. Transactions of the Orthopaedic Research Society. San Diego (CA); 2007.

80. Landesberg R, Takeuchi E, Puzas JE. Differential activation by cytokines of mitogen-activated protein kinases in bovine temporomandibular-joint disc cells. Arch Oral Biol 1999;44:41–8.

81. Sun WS, Moffat KL, Lu HH. Characterization of fibrochondrocytes derived from the ligament-bone insertion [abstract 0200]. Transactions of the Orthopaedic Research Society. San Diego (CA); 2007.

82. Fujioka H, Thakur R, Wang GJ, et al. Comparison of surgically attached and non-attached repair of the rat Achilles tendon-bone interface. Cellular organization and type X collagen expression. Connect Tissue Res 1998;37:205–18.

83. Grana WA, Egle DM, Mahnken R, et al. An analysis of autograft fixation after anterior cruciate ligament reconstruction in a rabbit model. Am J Sports Med 1994;22:344–51.

84. Kobayashi M, Watanabe N, Oshima Y, et al. The fate of host and graft cells in early healing of bone tunnel after tendon graft. Am J Sports Med 2005;33: 1892–7.

85. Wang IE, Shan J, Choi R, et al. Role of osteoblast-fibroblast interactions in the formation of the ligament-to-bone interface. J Orthop Res 2007;25:1609–20.

86. Jiang J, Nicoll SB, Lu HH. Co-culture of osteoblasts and chondrocytes modulates cellular differentiation in vitro. Biochem Biophys Res Commun 2005;338:762–70.

87. Shan JM, Wang IE, Lu HH. Osteoblast-fibroblast interactions modulate cell phenotypes through paracrine and autocrine regulations [abstract 0030]. Transactions of the Orthopaedic Research Society. San Diego (CA); 2007.

88. Lim JK, Hui J, Li L, et al. Enhancement of tendon graft osteointegration using mesenchymal stem cells in a rabbit model of anterior cruciate ligament reconstruction. Arthroscopy 2004;20:899–910.

89. Nawata K, Minamizaki T, Yamashita Y, et al. Development of the attachment zones in the rat anterior cruciate ligament: changes in the distributions of proliferating cells and fibrillar collagens during postnatal growth. J Orthop Res 2002; 20:1339–44.

90. Gao J, Messner K, Ralphs JR, et al. An immunohistochemical study of enthesis development in the medial collateral ligament of the rat knee joint. Anat Embryol (Berl) 1996;194:399–406.

91. French MM, Rose S, Canseco J, et al. Chondrogenic differentiation of adult dermal fibroblasts. Ann Biomed Eng 2004;32:50–6.

92. Nicoll SB, Wedrychowska A, Smith NR, et al. Modulation of proteoglycan and collagen profiles in human dermal fibroblasts by high density micromass culture and treatment with lactic acid suggests change to a chondrogenic phenotype. Connect Tissue Res 2001;42:59–69.

93. Vogel KG. The effect of compressive loading on proteoglycan turnover in cultured fetal tendon. Connect Tissue Res 1996;34:227–37.

94. Vogel KG, Ordog A, Pogany G, et al. Proteoglycans in the compressed region of human tibialis posterior tendon and in ligaments. J Orthop Res 1993;11:68–77.

95. Wang IE, Lu HH. Role of cell-cell interactions in the regeneration of soft tissue-to-bone interface. Proceedings of the IEEE Engineering Biology and Medicine Society 2006;1:783–6.

96. Dunn MG, Tria AJ, Kato YP, et al. Anterior cruciate ligament reconstruction using a composite collagenous prosthesis. A biomechanical and histologic study in rabbits. Am J Sports Med 1992;20:507–15.

97. Cooper JA, Sahota JS, Gorum WJ, et al. . Biomimetic tissue-engineered anterior cruciate ligament replacement. Proc Natl Acad Sci USA 2007;104:3049–54.

98. Spalazzi JP, Doty SB, Moffat KL, et al. Development of controlled matrix heterogeneity on a triphasic scaffold for orthopedic interface tissue engineering. Tissue Eng 2006;12:3497–508.

99. Spalazzi JP, Dagher E, Doty SB, et al. In vivo evaluation of a multiphased scaffold designed for orthopaedic interface tissue engineering and soft tissue-to-bone integration. J Biomed Mater Res 2008;86A:1–12.

100. Spalazzi JP, Moffat KL, Rodeo SA, et al. Design of a novel stratified scaffold for ACL-to-Bone interface tissue engineering. Transactions of the International Symposium on Ligaments and Tendons VIII. Stanford (CA); 2008. p. 40.

101. Spalazzi JP, Vyner MC, Jacobs MT, et al. Scaffold-induced compressive loading of tendon grafts promotes matrix remodeling and the expression of fibrocartilage-related markers. Clin Orthop Relat Res 2008;466(8):1938–48.

102. Khan SN, Bostrom MP, Lane JM. Bone growth factors. Orthop Clin North Am 2000;31:375–88.

103. Ramp WK, Dillaman RM, Lenz LG, et al. A serum substitute promotes osteoblast-like phenotypic expression in cultured cells from chick calvariae. Bone Miner 1991;15:1–17.

104. Lu HH, Kofron MD, El Amin SF, et al. In vitro bone formation using muscle-derived cells: a new paradigm for bone tissue engineering using polymer-bone morphogenetic protein matrices. Biochem Biophys Res Commun 2003; 305:882–9.

105. Kumagai J, Sarkar K, Uhthoff HK, et al. Immunohistochemical distribution of type I, II and III collagens in the rabbit supraspinatus tendon insertion. J Anat 1994;185(Pt 2):279–84.

106. Blevins FT, Djurasovic M, Flatow EL, et al. Biology of the rotator cuff tendon. Orthop Clin North Am 1997;28:1–16.

107. Gerber C, Schneeberger AG, Perren SM, et al. Experimental rotator cuff repair. A preliminary study. J Bone Joint Surg Am 1999;81:1281–90.

108. Rodeo SA. Biologic augmentation of rotator cuff tendon repair. J Shoulder Elbow Surg 2007;16:S191–7.

109. Iannotti JP, Codsi MJ, Kwon YW, et al. Porcine small intestine submucosa augmentation of surgical repair of chronic two-tendon rotator cuff tears. A randomized, controlled trial. J Bone Joint Surg Am 2006;88:1238–44.

110. Coons DA, Alan BF. Tendon graft substitutes-rotator cuff patches. Sports Med Arthrosc 2006;14:185–90.

111. Sclamberg SG, Tibone JE, Itamura JM, et al. Six-month magnetic resonance imaging follow-up of large and massive rotator cuff repairs reinforced with porcine small intestinal submucosa. J Shoulder Elbow Surg 2004;13:538–41.

112. Derwin KA, Baker AR, Spragg RK, et al. Commercial extracellular matrix scaffolds for rotator cuff tendon repair. Biomechanical, biochemical, and cellular properties. J Bone Joint Surg Am 2006;88:2665–72.

113. Inoue N, Ikeda K, Aro HT, et al. Biologic tendon fixation to metallic implant augmented with autogenous cancellous bone graft and bone marrow in a canine model. J Orthop Res 2002;20:957–66.

114. Yoshimoto H, Shin YM, Terai H, et al. A biodegradable nanofiber scaffold by electrospinning and its potential for bone tissue engineering. Biomaterials 2003;24:2077–82.

115. Garreta E, Gasset D, Semino C, et al. Fabrication of a three-dimensional nanostructured biomaterial for tissue engineering of bone. Biomol Eng 2007;24: 75–80.

116. Baker BM, Mauck RL. The effect of nanofiber alignment on the maturation of engineered meniscus constructs. Biomaterials 2007;28:1967–77.

117. Nerurkar NL, Elliott DM, Mauck RL. Mechanics of oriented electrospun nanofibrous scaffolds for annulus fibrosus tissue engineering. J Orthop Res 2007; 25:1018–28.

118. Li WJ, Danielson KG, Alexander PG, et al. Biological response of chondrocytes cultured in three-dimensional nanofibrous poly(epsilon-caprolactone) scaffolds. J Biomed Mater Res A 2003;67:1105–14.

119. Lee CH, Shin HJ, Cho IH, et al. Nanofiber alignment and direction of mechanical strain affect the ECM production of human ACL fibroblast. Biomaterials 2005;26: 1261–70.

120. Bashur CA, Dahlgren LA, Goldstein AS. Effect of fiber diameter and orientation on fibroblast morphology and proliferation on electrospun poly(D,L-lactic-co-glycolic acid) meshes. Biomaterials 2006;27:5681–8.

121. Ma Z, Kotaki M, Inai R, et al. Potential of nanofiber matrix as tissue-engineering scaffolds. Tissue Eng 2005;11:101–9.

122. Christenson EM, Anseth KS, van den Beucken JJ, et al. Nanobiomaterial applications in orthopedics. J Orthop Res 2007;25:11–22.

123. Pham QP, Sharma U, Mikos AG. Electrospinning of polymeric nanofibers for tissue engineering applications: a review. Tissue Eng 2006;12:1197–211.

124. Li WJ, Mauck RL, Cooper JA, et al. Engineering controllable anisotropy in electrospun biodegradable nanofibrous scaffolds for musculoskeletal tissue engineering. J Biomech 2007;40:1686–93.

125. Murugan R, Ramakrishna S. Design strategies of tissue engineering scaffolds with controlled fiber orientation. Tissue Eng 2007;13:1845–66.

126. Pham QP, Sharma U, Mikos AG. Electrospun poly(epsilon-caprolactone) microfiber and multilayer nanofiber/microfiber scaffolds: characterization of scaffolds and measurement of cellular infiltration. Biomacromolecules 2006;7: 2796–805.

127. Itoi E, Berglund LJ, Grabowski JJ, et al. Tensile properties of the supraspinatus tendon. J Orthop Res 1995;13:578–84.

128. Moffat KL, Levine WN, Lu HH. In vitro evaluation of rotator cuff tendon fibroblasts on aligned composite scaffold of polymer nanofibers and hydroxyapatite nanoparticles [abstract 1477]. Transactions of the Orthopaedic Research Society. San Diego (CA); 2008.

129. Jiang J, Leong NL, Mung J, et al. Interaction between zonal populations of articular chondrocytes suppresses chondrocyte mineralization and this process is mediated by PTHrP. Osteoarthritis Cartilage 2008;16:70–82.

Index

Note: Page numbers of article titles are in **boldface** type.

A

Achilles tendinopathy, chronic, platelet-rich-plasma in, 117–118, 119
Adenosine, 114
Allograft tissue, disinfection of, 133–135
    aseptic processing, ethylene oxide, gamma irradiation, and chemical soaking
      in, compared, 134
  preparation of, and processing of, 132–135
    specific processes for, 135–137
  processing of, new techniques in, **127–141**
  terminal sterilization and packaging of, 137
Allograft transplantation, for replacement of meniscus, 146–147
Allografts, bone and tissue, tissue banking and, 127
Amnesia, in concussion, 100, 101
Angiogenic modalities, skeletal muscle engineering with, 5–6
Anterior cruciate ligament, and bone interface tissue engineering, design considerations
  in, 158–160
  animal, injury of, response to, 54
  human, injury of, response to, 52–53
  injury of, clinical significance of, 51–52
    current treatment of, 51–52
    osteoarthritis after, 51, 52
    substitute scaffold in, in vitro development of, 55–56
  navigation of, and reconstruction of, current literature on, 42–44, 45
    overview of, 42, 43, 44
  non-union of, hypothesis for etiology of, 53, 54–55, 56
  primary repair of, biologic augmentation of, 57–58
    collagen-platelet composites in, 57–58
    current status and potential of, **51–62**
    future directions in, 58
    growth factors in, 57
    hyaluronic acid as scaffold treatment in, 57
    scaffolds in, 57
  reconstruction of, history of, 42
    incidence of, 41
    navigated knee stability examination in, 46–47
    navigated tunnel placement in, 44–46
    navigated versus conventional, clinical outcomes of, 47–48
    navigation of, 48, 49
Arthritis, replacement of meniscus and, 152

Clin Sports Med 28 (2009) 177–182
doi:10.1016/S0278-5919(08)00112-9
0278-5919/08/$ – see front matter © 2008 Elsevier Inc. All rights reserved.

sportsmed.theclinics.com

Moving?

Make sure your subscription moves with you!

To notify us of your new address, find your **Clinics Account Number** (located on your mailing label above your name), and contact customer service at:

E-mail: elspcs@elsevier.com

800-654-2452 (subscribers in the U.S. & Canada)
314-453-7041 (subscribers outside of the U.S. & Canada)

Fax number: 314-523-5170

Elsevier Periodicals Customer Service
11830 Westline Industrial Drive
St. Louis, MO 63146

* To ensure uninterrupted delivery of your subscription, please notify us at least 4 weeks in advance of move.

Printed and bound by CPI Group (UK) Ltd, Croydon, CR0 4YY

03/10/2024

01040444-0016